E

Personal Training Business

The 5 x 5 rule for working the hours you want and charging the fees you're worth

Chris Knott

Copyright © 2019 Chris Knott

ISBN: 978-1-6945-8813-5

DEDICATION

To my beautiful wife Kate, who fills my life with love and
laughter,
My dad Graham, who couldn't have been any more perfect as a
role model,
My mum Louisa, who cares for me unconditionally,
My sisters Lucy, Kelly & Jenny who inspire me to be a better
person,
And finally, to the best thing that ever happened to me, Indy.
You made dreams become a reality

We can live in a world that we design

CONTENTS

BUSINESS

DEVELOPMENT

FOREWARD
By Dan Reeve

Twenty years ago I walked into my first job within the fitness industry. Fresh out of university and PT school, I was ready to launch my enthusiasm and newly acquired knowledge onto anyone who would listen. I wanted to change the world, one squat and dumbbell press at a time. I read every training and nutrition article, magazine, and book going. This was long before social media, and fitness and health in general were far less prevalent than they are now.

Being an ex-professional athlete and looking the part, I quickly gained business and began my mission to help others become the best they could be. This worked incredibly well for me for over ten years. I travelled a lot and enjoyed everything London had to offer at the time. My work days often started before 5am and wouldn't end until after 9pm, consisting of eight or more training sessions, six days a week. Over this period of my life I easily took over 20,000 one-to-one PT sessions.

I was sensible enough to take a weekend break every so often, but my relationships and health suffered. I was more interested in taking sessions and earning money than personal development and in the end, I was burned out and left feeling purposeless and empty.

Over this period, I had clients who trained with me from day one. The only time clients left was when they moved away. My retention was excellent, but this was more through convenience and friendship than results and life change.

The other reason was because I never changed my prices. I charged £40-50 an hour in 2000 and the same in 2012. How many of my clients in Kensington and Chelsea had seen their house prices skyrocket by 30% or more in this time? How many had seen their annual salaries increase? Yet here I was doing the same thing, working the same hours for the same money.

I knew how to coach, I knew how to relate and be personable, but I didn't know how to run a business. I needed to learn how to grow, how and when to charge more, and when to cut hours or clients. I remember lecturing CEOs, lawyers, and bankers on the inner workings of the Krebs cycle and the biomechanics of the running gait to give credibility to my profession, and yet I had no clue how to earn more. When I needed to save for a holiday or house deposit, I simply worked more hours.

I'm sure parts of this story will ring true with a lot of you. The enthusiasm and genuine care to help people will only ever get us so far. There comes a point where you realise that all the knowledge about your subject and all the passion in the world won't pay the bills or really fulfil you.

After a year of travelling, education, soul searching, and re-defining my purpose and values, in 2013 I returned to the UK and the industry with a new plan. I had always worked hard but now it was time to work smart too, but most importantly, it was time to invest in myself properly. Then, in 2014 on a Charles Poliquin course in Marbella, Spain, I met Chris.

Since then I've watched Chris grow and grow, first from afar and then together at the FLF Performance Centre. He is meticulous with everything he does and leaves no stone unturned in pursuit of excellence. What I like most about Chris is his analytical nature. Like me, he loves numbers and systems, and *The 5 x 5 Rule* was born from his own success as a PT.

He came to understand personal training as a business in half the time it took me, with his insistence on working hard—but smart first. Whether it's lecturing in his seminars or conversing with industry legends on his podcast, Chris always delivers amazing content and wisdom. With *The 5 x 5 Rule*, he hasn't tried to reinvent the wheel by telling trainers how to coach a deadlift or understand a calorie deficit. Instead, has built systems to attend a neglected but critical part of this sector: the business side of personal training.

Today I sit here boxing clever. I have systems in place to support all aspects of a multi-faceted business. I have a new sense of my own significance and understand that my time is worth something. I love coaching and will never stop, but now

I do it at the times I want, with the clients I want, and at a price my experience, education, and the economy set. A lot of this comes from the lessons learned from regular chats with Chris.

This book isn't just important; it's essential. It's a must-read for all PI's and coaches who need to learn how to supply a better service for their clients and enhance, prolong, and give structure to their career. Adding these critical elements into your business and daily habits will dramatically improve how you operate. Now settle in, grab a pen and paper, and reap the benefits of *The 5 x 5 Rule*.

Affamato Come Un Lupo

INTRODUCTION

Being self-employed can be both a blessing and a curse. You can work when you want, how you want, and for how much you want in a field that matches your passion and expertise. It's a way of living your dream and breaking free from the restrictions that come with working for someone else. If you want to live life on your own terms, it pays to be your own employer—but it comes at a cost.

When you work for a company, although they dictate your hours, pay, and development, your security lies in their hands. You trade freedom for peace of mind. You know that if you turn up at your delegated times, do your designated jobs, and interact amicably with your colleagues, you'll be rewarded with a consistent income. Working for a company also means you don't have to worry about factors such as doing your own tax, marketing, and business models. You simply turn up, do your job, and leave the running of the corporation to the big cats upstairs. You may not live your life by your own design, but if you stay with the company long enough, hit their targets, and turn up with a smile on your face, you may get a promotion or an increase in pay every now and again. You have much less to worry about and a safety net to fall back on. You get holidays, sick days, and can plan your life around a rigid working structure. It's a tangible existence for many. The problem is when companies capitalise on passion. They're aware that their employees love the field that they're in, so know that finances may not be the primary drive. In no industry is this more prevalent than the world of fitness.

Being a personal trainer is great. You get to wear your gym kit to work, socialise in a relaxed environment, train as much as you want, and help people look and feel better about themselves. It's an extremely rewarding job that is easy immerse yourself in. With the plethora of information so readily available online, you can grow your skill set every day.

It's an exciting time to be a coach and with so many people looking to get fit and healthy, it's safe to say that the demand for professional, diligent trainers will always be there. This being said, there is an unfortunate reality to the world of personal training that many overlook. The personal training industry has one of the highest drop-out rates of any profession. It's estimated that the average career span of a PT is around eighteen months, with common reasons for leaving being poor pay and working unsociable hours. If you work for a chain gym, you'll always have a glass ceiling when it comes to income. Sure, you don't have to pay rent and always have access to a high stream of members, but your earnings will always be heavily syphoned by the company you work for. If you go self-employed, you're suddenly not just a personal trainer anymore; you're a salesman, marketer, accountant, content developer, and finally, a business owner. The problem is, we don't get taught about any of these things during our personal training education.

In the summer 2009, I had a phone call with a personal training company about doing one of their intense seven-week qualifications. I had decided that after one year of studying sports and exercises sciences at university, I wanted to get out into the world and earn money instead of increasing my student debts. I remember sitting on the fence for a little bit, unsure about whether or not it was the right decision, until the person on the other end of the phone uttered those fateful words: "You can earn anything from £30-40,000 a year as a PT." That made up my mind right there and then. I got off the phone, elated like I'd just won the lottery. With both naivety and exuberance, I informed my friends that I'd just made a thorough and astute decision to become a personal trainer and that I'd be earning around £35,000 a year. Or so I thought.

Maths can't lie. If you crunch some numbers and set realistic targets, you start to see a business plan appear. If the average cost of a personal training session is £30 an hour (which it was back in 2009, but bizarrely is still now), you would need to do 1167 sessions a year to earn £35,000. Taking into account four weeks off for holidays and Christmas, delivering twenty-five sessions per week over forty-eight weeks of the year would make this target feasible. So, was the coach I spoke to telling the truth? Well, it depends.

First, you have to account for building up your business to a position where you're delivering twenty-five sessions per week. To do this, you need to build a brand and a reputation for being good at what you do. It took me five years from qualifying to get up to twenty-five sessions a week. I had to build my confidence, experience, plus sales and marketing skills to reach this point. It wasn't easy and I struggled a lot.

Second, you have to look at how much of that £35,000 you take home. The average rent at an independent gym is £500 a month. Therefore, you immediately have to subtract £6,000 per annum off your income. You could work in a commercial gym and so subsidise your rent, but this means dropping your hourly earnings to around £15 an hour. If you wanted to earn £35,000 a year in that scenario, you'd need to be doing forty-nine sessions a week, which isn't ideal. Many people wouldn't scoff at taking home £29,000 a year being self-employed and doing a job they love, but again, this notion holds a sobering reality. Client cancellations, seasonal variance in PT uptake, and the often-overlooked fluctuations in your own confidence and ability to sign up new clients will all impact your income. I wasn't hitting a gross income of over £30,000 until year seven of being a personal trainer. The key idea here is *gross* income. To get to a point where I was busy and happy with the amount of money I was charging, I invested into my on-going education—a lot. If you account for books, courses, online content, and all forms of CPD, I was spending a sizeable sum on further development. You could argue it had its perks from a deductible tax expense perspective, but this wasn't practical for my own personal income and savings. I could technically say I was earning £30,000 a year, but my business wasn't making that much—far from it. When I assessed my finances and looked at how much money was left over after all business expenses were paid, I would have only been able to pay myself around £17,000 a year. After seven years, I was still technically on minimum wage. Something had to give.

Things started to change over the next three years. Instead of just tracking my income, I started to assess it. I stopped looking at gross income and more at net. I started to design business models and look how I could earn more in other areas. I made peace with my desire to work for passion and instead realised that I owed it to myself to start earning real money. I began to have a deliberate plan of action and as a result, things started to change. My mindset altered and I realised that as great as it was being a personal trainer, I'd always be frustrated if I didn't value my time and look to grow my business. After a substantial period in the industry, the penny dropped. Not only *can* you combine your passion with a deliberate, intelligent business model, but you *should* do it as well. The more you earn, the better your services get. The better your services get, the more people who'll want to do business with you. It has a snowball effect.

Suddenly the emotional attachment had been dropped. I stopped caring as much about whether I offended people with what I was charging and started to care more about whether I hit the weekly, monthly, and yearly goals that I set myself. It was a turning point in my career and one that coincided with getting together with my now wife, Kate. I realised that there would come a time where working every hour of the day on a gym floor was neither practical nor wise. This was the conception of the 5 x 5 rule.

If there was one thing I was definitely guilty of in my early years as a PT, it was working haphazardly. I didn't have set hours or a set goal; I just worked whenever I thought I should. If someone wanted me to train them at a time, I would. As PTs, we're martyrs to our work and often accommodate anyone at any time. Being with my wife made me respect my weekends and evenings again. It made me re-think how I wanted to spend my time and how I could alter my business model so it worked for me, not against me. The 5 x 5 rule is a business model that describes how to work five days a week doing five sessions a day. You regain your weekends and evenings if you're astute with your booking system. It's a way of changing your schedule so you get to do a job you love while also having a life outside of work—but it doesn't stop there.

If you work for a company, you have the prospect of earning more via promotions and loyalty. The longer you work, the more money you should get paid. This is the way it should be in personal training as well. The problem is, most personal trainers are never taught how to do this. They're not taught about business models, how to increase fees, and how to plan long term. In this book, we'll explore how you can incrementally increase your hourly rate so that your earnings are proportional to your time in the industry. Instead of working more to earn more, you charge more to earn more. The 5 x 5 rule teaches you how to increase your fees by a minimum of 25% per hour over a five-year timeline.

Finally, we look at expansion. This book provides details on how you can build your brand, online presence, and multiple forms of income through maximising time efficiency and sticking to a business model. It has deliberate, proven methods specific to the world of personal training. My goal is that you learn from my experiences. I want you to fast track the years of frustration I had and be able to create a service that is as beneficial to the general public as it is profitable for you. This book was written by a personal trainer, for personal trainers. I wrote each chapter and posted it in a private Facebook forum for a group of fifty coaches with a variety of experience and qualifications. The topics featured are based on my own experiences and what the members of the group requested to read about. By using this method, I believe I have put together the most relevant and applicable information that PTs need to learn. It's far from a quick fix, as it will take a lot of patience and effort, but if you carry out all these teachings consistently, there is no reason why you can't surpass £40,000 net profit (after expenses) by your fifth year in the industry. Actions speak louder than words. So read this book, apply it to your own model, and create a formidable business in a field you love.

BUSINESS

THE BASICS

Picture the scene: I was chatting to a client in between sets. We were stood next to the pendulum squat, him telling me about Liverpool's recent resurgence in form. It's 9:55pm. I started work at 5:30am. I'd love to say he was my twelfth client of the day, that I'd been back to back since dawn, but unfortunately, this wasn't the case. He was my fifth client, and my first client the next day was at 6am. For most of you reading this, you'll think, "Yep, been there, done that." It's a personal trainer's rite of passage to work stupid, ungodly hours. But why?

The answer is clear. First, it's about money. We don't want to pass on the opportunity to earn. Second, it's being accommodating. We want to make sure we fit around the client's schedule, not them around ours. Why else would we be in the gym at 10pm after almost sixteen hours of being there?

How do you break the mould? How do you go from over worked and under paid to working on your own accord for money that justifies your efforts? This is something we're not taught on personal training certifications. I got qualified, started training people, then just had to figure the rest out. I wasn't taught about business, finances, or even how to conduct a sales transaction. I was green and it led to frustration. My biggest mistake was assuming that I'd make a lot of money simply being good at what I do. Unfortunately, this is only half of the equation.

I would say there are universal rules for business that translate to any profession. It doesn't matter whether you're selling PT sessions, clothes, or ice cream: you need to establish who wants to buy your product, how you to reach them, how you make them want to buy your product, then how to increase your profit margins. It's a step by step process, with each commodity supplying objective data that can be assessed, reviewed, and addressed. A deficiency in one area leads to a weakness in the whole chain, and then your business suffers.

The thing is, being good at sales doesn't make you good at business. Just as long-term weight loss is a holistic process of diet, lifestyle, training, and mindset manipulation, so too is building a successful brand. You must assess all areas. Even if someone can sell sand to the Arabs, can they track their finances, plan for growth, retain their clientele, and get results? It's not just about money and transactions; it's about creating systems that may one day let you sell your business.

How much time do you work on your business? This doesn't mean studying, check ins, or social media. These are "in-business" commodities that enhance or deliver the product. They're things that could be done in free time or even subsidised. I'm talking about planning for growth, assessing finances, reviewing where you're losing time and money, and how you could tidy up loose ends. They're the things that you, the business owner, should care about the most. As this is your brand, your money, your assets, and essentially your life's work. You want to know which direction it's going.

When Richard Branson goes into a meeting, what do you think he wants to know? Do you think they spend a lot of time dwelling on train times and staff training? On the other hand, how much time do you think they spend talking about monthly financial projections, profit margins, marketing strategies, brand development, company ethos, and competitors? These business factors are essential to assess for growth. If you don't even know them, never mind address them, how successful do you think your business is likely to be?

Let's say you've decided that after ten years in the business, you want to give up personal training, raise some money, and live the good life out on a farm detached from reality. The thing is, you have clients (both in person and online), a brand, and a reputation. You wouldn't want ten years of early starts, late finishes, educational courses, networking, and hard work to be in vain. You should at least be able to gain some financial reward for your efforts. The question is, how much is your business worth?

Imagine you're sitting in a coffee shop across the table from me. I am a millionaire business owner looking to acquire independent personal training businesses in order to consolidate a client base of a hundred or more before opening a new gym facility in the area. Could you sell your business to me, and for how much?

Is this a question you've ever thought about before? If not, take some time to close the book, have a think, and write stuff down. How much money would you want for someone to buy your business, and how would you justify it? Remember, businessmen are shrewd and they'll be able to smell weakness. If you can't validate how much you're asking for, then they aren't going to buy off you. What would you say?

"I've invested this much into my education."
"I have this many social media followers."
"I've worked sixteen-hour days every day for the past five years."

These points may be noble of you to say, but it's largely irrelevant. In fact, the investor won't care about that at all. They'll want to know about financial growth, profit margins, lead generation, retention/uptake, and scaling your brand. As soon as you stray away from these areas, they'll lose interest. They appreciate that time is money and that they aren't going to want to invest in this venture. If you want to assess and grow your business, you need to know the following commodities like the back of your hand.

Financial Growth

What were you charging one year ago? How much have you increased your rates by in the past twelve months and what factors have led to this increase? Was it education? Results? Improvement in reputation? What have you done that you can then replicate that has led to justifying charging (or making) more money? Can you then present this, week by week, month by month, in clear objective data? Where are your stats?

Profit Margins

How much do you make per session? Not charge per session but make per session. This is your gym rent divided by how many sessions you do per month, subtracted from your hourly rate. You can even go one further and factor in daily commute costs to get a true figure:

Monthly delivery: 80 sessions
Gym rent: £500
Cost per session: 500/80 = £6.25
Cost in petrol per day: £5
Average sessions per day: 4
Cost of commute per session: £1.25
Total cost per session: £7.50
Average hourly rate: £40
Average profit per hour: £32.50
Profit Percentage: £32.50/£40 x 100 = 81.25%

How is this number affected by losing a client or a client going on holiday? Has this number increased or decreased in the past 6–12 months? What could you do to improve this number, whether it be paying less rent, reducing commute costs, or increasing fees?

Lead Generation

How many enquiries do you get per month? Where do they come from? How much time do you have to invest in each mode in order to retain this rate of enquiry? Do you have to spend money on marketing or advertising to do so? If so, how much does it cost and is it warranted? Are you spending too much time on an area that doesn't validate it, for example social media, when enquiries are low? Do you have a formula that is replicable for generating leads, be it online or in person?

Uptake/Retention

What is your conversion rate like based on lead generation? How long do you have to spend on the gym floor or online to generate ten leads? Out of these, how many sign up? Do you have a system that is making your uptake in products more successful? This could be taster sessions, the way you present your packages, the quality of your consultations, and making sure you're sitting down with the right people in the first place.

When people sign up with you, how long are they committing? What is the net spend per client? Do you send them questionnaires asking them about customer service, what they're happy with, and what they'd improve? Do you know why they are leaving? Could you improve factors that are leading to people not using your services anymore? What are the main factors that keep people training with you? How do you enhance these factors? Do you have periods where you go quiet due to the holidays? When is your busiest time? How do you periodise your busiest times so you can maximise your efforts in generating leads? So, for example, doing a heavy marketing campaign in November so you have emails and contact numbers ready for a push in uptake come January/February.

Scaling Your Business/Brand Development

If your goal is to work as a trainer, do you have systems in place to grow your reputation, increase fees, and work less and on your own terms? How does your business grow and become scalable? Will you eventually employ people to work for you? Will you eventually have a passive product? How do you periodise yourself out of the business so that you're working *on* projects and not *in* projects? Will you have the same role you do now in five years' time? Do you have a five-year plan at all?

Taking all of these into account, what if your answer to the initial question sounded like this?

I currently deliver an average of twenty-two sessions per week between the hours of 7am to 1pm Monday to Friday. This average has been calculated over the past six months. My average hourly rate has increased by 25% from £40 to £50 in the past twenty-four months. As I pay £500 a month in rent per month, I currently make £44.32 per session, which is a profit of 88.6%. This has increased by 18.6% from 70% in the past twelve months. I would attribute my growth to getting better results with my clients, leading to an increase in word of mouth referrals. I invest 5% of my monthly earnings into education, with the most useful and applicable course being the one I attended in biomechanics. I attribute my skills as a trainer growing to this course so am going to focus on more courses in this area so that it becomes my niche.

I post on social media five times a week and currently have a following of 5,000 people on Instagram. I use Instagram the most as this is the avenue which I gain the most interactions and enquiries. If I post five times a week, I get on average five enquiries for my online services per week. Three out of the twenty monthly enquires sign up, which means my average growth for my online business is three new clients per month. My online services cost £100 a month and I have a capacity of twenty clients for quality control.

Based on my current figures, my average monthly income is £5,900. My goal is to increase one-to-one session rates to £55 in the next twelve months but also drop my gym floors to three days a week, delivering six sessions a day Monday, Wednesday, and Friday. This would mean I earn the same amount of money from one-to-one PT but only work three days instead of five. In the same timeframe, I would like to increase online fees to £120 per month. Working two days less means I can increase my online client base from twenty to thirty, enhancing my monthly income to £7,560. This is a 28% growth in income in twelve months with no increase in outgoings.

As all my figures are based off averages that account for seasonal variance, my annual before tax gross income is currently £70,800. I have set systems in place for client screenings, questionnaires, diet plans, FAQs, programme design, online support, online forums, and payments, all which could be taught to another coach. Given that I continue with the same strategies I have in place now, my projection for the next three years is that my annual income will grow by 8% per year. This equates £230,000 generated in that time. If you were to buy my current business, plus my three-year model, I would value it at £250,000, as you will have funds to subsidise work and invest more in marketing.

Sound farfetched? It might in the world of personal training as interactions like this are rare, if existent at all. However, conversations like this will happen thousands of times a day in the world of business management. It's about acquiring assets, investing, and validating spending based on a sound business model. Want to turn your personal training job into a business? This book will tell you how.

MANAGING YOUR FINANCES

Profit and loss are the backbones of business. I spent years being incredibly frustrated that I was over working and under charging; however, I never did the maths to see what I needed to work on. I used to think that charging more would lead to a better quality of life. It does, without a doubt, but it's the last piece in the financial jigsaw puzzle. First you need to lay foundations and establish a starting point for your model. In business, you need to account for the worst possible situation. It sounds a little pessimistic, but in doing so you'll avoid being in high pressure situations or getting desperate. Ever gotten nervous about having to pay your rent and house bills at the end of the month? I have and it's not nice. Here are some strategies to prevent that from happening.

Figure out every single penny you spend a month. This needs to be everything you are accountable to pay for: gym rent, car, petrol, phone, bills, mortgage. If your records stretch back far enough, find your average spends over the past 3–6 months. Times this figure by 1.2. This somewhat arbitrary figure accounts for a 20% excess of spending for any unexpected bills or events. You can increase to 25–30% if you feel cautious. If your outgoings are £1,500 a month, your new figure is £1,800 (20% increase). Divide this figure by the amount you charge per hour. For example, if you charge £35, then $1800/35 = 51$. This is the number of sessions you need to deliver per month to break even. You now know that thirteen sessions per week covers your basic overheads ($51/4$). As long as you hit this many sessions a week, you break even, and that's is essential. Regardless of how much you manage to increase your earnings by, I would highly recommend you take the following advice: "Treat the money that you earn like it's not your money." I have been a personal trainer for ten years now. If I've seen one clear trend, it's that you have a rise and fall in sales from month to month. Usually the increase and decline are proportional to each other, so a good month financially will be followed by a quiet one, but be busier with one-to-one sessions due to the number of people you signed up. Long story short, there are highs and lows. If you are a PT new to the industry, take solace in the fact that undulating income is completely normal. Things are never linear. It is completely possible for your income to be £800 one month and £3,500 the next. Holidays, jobs, and family responsibilities will delay people in up-taking PT, yet when all these things fall into alignment, you suddenly have an influx of people signing up. You need to view yourself as a business, not a sole trader. Draw money out of your account once per month and learn how to live with it. Doing so will teach you a valuable lesson about money and business.

Imagine it's the last week of the month. You have £300 in your bank account and your £500 gym rent is due in four days. You are worried that you won't be able to afford rent and may have to approach the gym owner where you work and explain the situation. Two days before the end of the month you get an inquiry and low and behold, they sign up. They buy ten sessions for £350 and save you for that month. You get out of jail this time, but don't want to make it a regular occurrence. But what if this person had been difficult and wanted a deal? What if they had offered you £300, take it or leave it? What would you have done?

To prevent situations like this, you need to learn how to be disciplined during your good months, not your bad ones. When you have an influx of cash, don't go out and spend it.

Leave it in your bank account and remember that it's not your money—it belongs to your business. Once you learn how to differentiate between your own spending and your business' spending, you will see an exponential improvement in the way you manage your business. Why? Because being on a wage makes you work harder. The best thing about it is that you're working hard for a company that you own. Every six months you could increase your own wage by a percentage proportional to how much your business has grown, allowing you to reap the rewards of your hard work. You get to give yourself a raise.

I'm a big believer that people treat you in a similar manner to the way you act. I think that transactions speak volumes about you as a business and what you're about. Taking a wad of scrunched up ten-pound notes doesn't exactly scream professionalism. The punter will assume this is just a means of you earning a bit of cash here and there. It's not a business or career. Sending people PDF and PayPal invoices or allowing them to pay via a card reader, on the other hand, shows that you're a legitimate business. If you want to be treated with respect, you need to behave in a formal manner.

Something I couldn't recommend enough is compartmentalising your income and delegating different pots to different aspects of your life. It takes a lot of discipline and organisation, but honestly, if you nail this part of your business, you'll massively reduce your financial stresses. This method is something I wish I'd done a lot longer ago. First let me ask you a question: If a course or seminar comes up you wish to attend, how do you know if you can afford to go or not? Is it by how much is in your account now? Is it how close it is to the end of the month when bills are due? Is it seasonal when you know clients will be away and work will be quiet? Personally, I don't think that investing in your education should have anything to do with any of these things. If you are like me, you love learning. However, the number of times I've made my life difficult for myself by going on a course I couldn't technically afford is scary. I was guilty of this in my younger years when my outgoings were low, but once my responsibilities changed, I needed a different strategy. Further learning is a direct investment in the growth of your own business. Therefore, the money that you spend on courses can be reclaimed as a tax-deductible expense. This means that if you're running your business as if you have a set wage, you don't have to eat into your own wage to pay for the course. This is ideal, as it doesn't impact the quality of your personal life.

Remember, you work for you. You are self-employed, meaning you are employed by yourself. You pay your own wages and when you work hard to earn money for the business, you are the benefactor—no one else. This is an important mantra. As I've said before, you must know what your average outgoings are as both an individual and a business. Differentiating between what you need to live and need to work is important. Here's an example:

Personal Outgoings
Mortgage/House rent
Phone bill
Council Tax
Car/Home insurance
Food
Weekend spends allowance

For most people this will range from anywhere between £1,500-2,500. It will depend on your age, whether you have children, and other personal responsibilities. Therefore, to make your life manageable, the wage that you pay yourself needs to be around x1.25 this figure, or £2,500 if your outgoings are £2,000 on average. The 25% increase is to factor in unexpected bills, occasional meals out, and just to give yourself to leeway when it comes to living. Now let's consider business outgoings.

<u>Business Outgoings</u>
Gym rent
Website hosting
Online consulting hosting (Zoom)
Online coaching
Commuting costs
CPD subscriptions (Audible, educational website fees, etc.)

Business outgoings, unlike personal outgoings, are tax deductible. If you're unsure about what you can and can't claim back on, be sure to speak to your accountant. It's only a natural progression that as your business grows, so will your business expenses. Therefore, it's important to pay attention to what you spend and why and know where you can be saving money on tax. Let's discuss how you can make your own life a lot easier for yourself using spreadsheets, analytics, and discipline.

If a trainer charges £35 and does 100 sessions a month, they earn £3,500. If their personal monthly outgoings are £1,250, then they may opt to pay themselves a wage out of their business of £1,750 a month. This is to cover all their *personal* outgoings. Therefore 50% (£1,750/£3,500) has now been accounted for as a wage. The rest is what's left to pay your business expenses (see business outgoings list). The more you can get these under control, the more you can astutely plan for education in the future. I created my own finance tracker by noting every single transaction that I made for my business and personal life. It sounds arduous, but it's quite easy. Open a spreadsheet and create three tabs: one for income, one for personal outgoings, and one for business outgoings. Every time you make a transaction, both in and out of your account, make a note in the appropriate tab. You can review your online bank statements at the same time each week and sift through all the cash flow. Here you'll see where your money's going and the state of your finances. I'd recommend doing this at the same time each week to create a habit.

At the end of each month, you'll have three extremely valuable pieces of information: total earnings, total personal outgoings, and total business expenses. You'll be able to see what you spend your money on and why you're not saving as much as you think. If your personal expenses are exceeding your set wage (£1,750), you know you are spending too much in that department. Therefore, you know you'll have to cut back on personal expenses the following month. Variance is a big factor here. You'll have set monthly direct debits for essentials you can't cut back on. Things like phones, running water, and commuting fees are unavoidable. However, meals out, clothes, and other accessories must be kept within your means if you want your business to thrive. A lot of personal trainers get frustrated by not having enough money, but this is only because they're not paying attention to where their money goes. Using a tracking system like this will let you know how much you'll be able to spend the following month. As soon as you learn to live within your wage, the financial magic starts to happen. Your biggest business expense will almost always be your gym rent. Factoring this in, the lower you keep monthly outgoings, the more you have to either save or reinvest in your business. Treat business expenses the same as you do with your personal expenses. Monitor them precisely and keep them as low as possible. There's an extremely important reason for this. Take a look at the following.

	Income	Business Exp.	Personal Exp.	Savings
Amount	£3,500	£850	£1,750	£900

Say this is a personal trainer's final P & L sheet for a month. They've taken £3,500 in earnings, spent £850 on business commodities, and delegated £1,750 as a wage. This would technically leave them with £900 to reinvest in the business for CPD or simply to save. The only problem here is that we've forgotten an incredibly important factor: tax. Taxes are scary for the self-employed. If you're not smart about putting money away, you can be left with some large tax bills that you have no other option to pay. This is why, come rain or shine, I recommend always putting away 20% of your monthly earnings for tax purposes. It's easy to assume you have money to spend, but when you take tax into consideration, your actual reinvest fund looks like this:

	Income	Tax	Business Exp.	Personal Exp.	Savings
Amount	£3,500	£700	£850	£1,750	£200

Suddenly paying all that money for a CPD course doesn't seem so wise. Businesses do not spend when their income stream doesn't warrant an investment, but personal trainers do. It's what makes us our own worst enemies and what leads to the over-qualified, under-paid frustration. You need to learn to be extremely disciplined with your money but also see where it's going and how much you can spend on what. Remember, the more you earn, the more you learn. Education is essential as a personal trainer, but CPD can't be prioritised over the financial wellbeing of a business. It must to earned through sales and profit margins.

The longer you track your monthly outgoings, the more valid your monthly averages will be. For example, twelve months of data is more reliable than three months. This way you can predict how long it will take you to save for something in a much more accurate manner. The biggest mistake I used to make was buying or investing in something just because the money was there. It may be in your account, but can you spend it? I'd hate to think that coaches out there panic and face scary repercussions for not factoring tax when self-employed. It's something I wish I had learned when doing my initial course. As a self-employed personal trainer, you'll be exempt on the personal allowance of your annual earnings (for the tax year 2019/20 this is £12,500, but this changes annually). You'll be taxed 20% on any money you declare over this amount up to the higher rate band. Therefore, taking the 2018/19 tax year as a guide, if you say you've earned £20,000 that year, you'll pay £1,500 in tax and national insurance of £1,509.76. You may be thinking, if I'm getting cash in hand, why would I want to pay more tax? First, if you ever intend to get on the property ladder, the bank will look at what you've declared over the past three years. If it's between the £16-20,000 a year mark, the most you're likely to get loaned to you is around £65,000. This won't get you much these days. You could always keep renting your flat, but renting is dead money. You also need to factor in having a family and bringing up kids someday. Could you do this where you live now?

If you're staying as a sole trader, it's incredibly important you put 20% aside each month for tax purposes. It's an essential part of business. You can't pick and choose when you'd like to be legitimate. I've known many a personal trainer who've been stung by this. Furthermore, remember the initial question: could you sell me your business? If this investor did put in an offer, do you think he'd want to see your official accounts? Absolutely, and you need to be consistent. Declare your money, set money aside for tax purposes, and invest in a good accountant. If you were to turn your business into a limited company, your wages come off your profit and loss. In other words, they're a tax-deductible expense. Therefore, if you pay yourself a wage, in a way it comes off your tax bill. You still get taxed as a payee, but it won't be much if you don't pay yourself a lot. Confused? Don't worry; I'll explain.

Let's say a PT is doing very well and earns £50,000 a year. If you are a sole trader, the total tax and national insurance you would pay based on the 2019/20 tax figures is £12,464.16— OUCH! You want to buy a house and so need to show you're earning. What do you do? Take the tax on the chin? Look to borrow the money? Keep living at your parents' house? Solution: set up as a limited company. When you are a limited company, the tax policy changes. If you have made a £50,000 profit, you would then take a minimal salary, say £12,500, and the corporation tax you would pay is £7,023. This leaves with company reserves of £29,943, part of which could be declared as a dividend, which currently holds a tax rate of 7.5% (the first £2,000 at 0%). Say you take a dividend of £25,000, plus your salary of £12,500. Now you would pay personal tax of £2,114.16.

Sole Trader total tax = £12,464 tax a year

Ltd Company total tax (including personal) = £9,137 tax a year

That's a completely legitimate way of paying £3,327 less tax per year if you track your earnings and have a good accountant. You don't have to let cash payments go missing and it gives you a much better chance of getting on the property ladder. Think long term: just because you don't intend to do something now doesn't mean you won't want to do it in the future. Not only does becoming a limited company scream professionalism, it means you must live within the wage you pay yourself as well. Everything becomes more official. You own a company and you're the boss. You can withdraw significant funds in dividends every three to six months. The tax has been accounted for and you now can spend on your family worry free. If your goal is to be in this industry for a long time and you intend to make a lot of money, becoming a limited company is definitely something I'd consider.

REDUCING LOSS

The Peppermint Tea Effect

Although increasing income gets a lot of the limelight, you can't neglect the fact the you can increase your profit margins by reducing outgoings. It doesn't make sense to stress the need to charge more money per hour if you're flippant with your spending. You're just losing money you've worked hard to gain. Tracking your outgoings is essential and having a date with your accounts would be advisable on a monthly, fortnightly, or even weekly basis. You need to see where all your money is going and whether it's justified or not. As the old saying goes, if you're not assessing, you're guessing. Scratching your head and wondering why you struggle to pay rent each month is nonsensical if you have no idea what your spending habits are like. Track every single penny you spend for one month. The results will scare you.

A standard coffee these days is around £2.50. If you grab one on your way to work and you work five days a week, you spend £50 on coffee a month. If you grab two a day, this goes to £100. Problems may also arise when you consider "subliminal" spends when you grab your coffee. How often do you grab a gluten-free brownie or other snack due to delivering five sessions back to back and being low on energy and blood sugar? This £2.50 then becomes £4.50. You may think nothing of it, but untracked spending will probably amount to £250 a month. If your monthly earnings average around £3,500, that's 7% of your income eaten away due to lack of planning. Cutting down spends isn't being cheap or tight, it's business sense. If you still can't see this, think of things like this. Tomorrow, you have to go in and increase all your clients' session prices by £2.50 per hour. How would you feel about this? Would you feel nervous? Scared? Like it wasn't warranted? The truth is, the idea of increasing your rates is one of the biggest psychological obstacles a PT will face. However, there is no difference (financially speaking) in increasing your hourly rate and cutting down your daily spends. From a profit and loss perspective, maths is maths. Real profit margins start to appear when you learn how to maximise both.

Like many PTs, I am a fiend for coffee. I'd comfortably spend anywhere from £2.50-£5 a day to get my fix. In my session delivery heyday, I'd think nothing of doing 6–7 sessions back to back with no breaks and no food. What got me through? That's right: copious amounts of caffeine. I'd have 2–3 cups a day, ranging from the gym's own supply to being brought one externally by a friendly colleague. Not only did this habit put a big dent in my bank balance, it was all having a negative impact on my health as well. My sleep suffered and with the early starts and long days, I was in the vicious cycle of becoming caffeine dependant. Something had to change as both my health and income was declining. Then I found a solution.

I needed to ween myself off caffeine. I also needed to cut back on spends. Then one day I grabbed a bag of peppermint tea from a local convenience shop. The box of twenty bags cost £2.50, the price of just one coffee. That meant an instant monthly saving of nearly £50. Wow! One small change can make a huge difference. The best thing about it is that tea bags can be reused when you fill up with hot water. It's not as strong, but the taste is still there. A lot of the time it's not necessarily the coffee that you want, it's just having something to drink. It's the habit more than anything. This prompts me to ask you, how can you use the peppermint tea effect on your spending? Where are you haphazardly spending money? Do you even know? This is why I believe it's essential to assess your bank statements on a regular basis. You'll notice small fees here and there that have been going out for months unnoticed. Maybe they were only for £7.99, which doesn't seem like much, but they add up in time. You can take this one step further by seeing what you spend your money on regularly and where you can make savings. Amazon has an awesome service called "Subscribe & Save" where you get 15% off each item if you subscribe to five items per month. If you get your supplements online or even some bulk foods such as oats and rice, you can make a great monthly saving simply by ordering it all together. A few clicks of a button managed to save me £40 on protein powder a month buying the same brand and amount. Remember, these small amounts of money leaking from your business could be contributing to saving up for a house, holiday, or wedding. You're making a rod for your own back by not taking simple steps to assess your spends. With some diligent tracking, discipline, and smart saving strategies, you could improve your profit and loss by £300-500 a month on a regular basis.

Although your gym rent is a set commodity, you can change the way you view it by using certain strategies. What I would do is set aside 2–3 months of gym rent when I have a good month. It sounds somewhat pessimistic, but trust me, it makes a big difference to financial pressures. Preparing in advance like this means come good month or bad month, your outlook is neutral. Your wage is your wage and it doesn't change.

Say you have a great month where you have an influx of new clients. You get three new people buy blocks of sessions along with your usual renewals. You usually average around £3,000 but this month you've done an amazing £4,750. You feel like you've cracked it. You're finally getting somewhere. I know the feeling: it's exciting, it's new, and you feel proud of yourself. It's during times like this the temptation to spend can be high. Whether it's on education, supplements, clothes, or other goods, you may think you have a surplus amount of income to enjoy.

An influx in client sign ups means that your following month will be high in delivery. When session delivery increases, your ability to generate income reduces. You will be spending your time in your business, not working on it. Instead of spending it, take the extra money you earned that month and set it aside in a different bank account. This account is purely for paying your rent. Getting ahead of yourself when it comes to paying rent is a business masterstroke. It keeps your spending at bay but most importantly, it stops you from worrying about money and just scraping by. Whenever you have a spike in earnings one month, your first port of call should be to set the money aside and accumulate at least 1–2 months of gym rent in savings. Doing so will reduce the likelihood of ever feeling desperate.

It's easy to become slack with your pricing structures when you have client asking for a deal, especially if it's been a quiet month for you. One of the biggest psychological components you'll encounter when it comes to increasing your fees is worrying about people paying it. If you know your rent is accounted for, this worry eases. Organising your finances is a critical part of financial growth. You must lay the foundations to give yourself the greatest chance of success. Without these fundamentals, growth will always be guess work and hope. This should never be the case. If you're happy in your gym and know you'll be working there for at least the next three months, negotiate with the gym owner to see if you can get 10–20% off your rent if you pay in advance. The percentage you ask for will depend on your negotiation skills, but even a 10% discount saves you £50 a month. This could go to a house bill or be set aside for savings for Christmas. Regardless of what you do with it, it's a simple way of positively impacting your P & L. The worst your gym owner can say is no, but they'll probably admire your business savviness. Whenever I wanted to increase my hourly rate for new clients, I did it during a phase when my gym rent had been paid upfront. If the person didn't sign up, what's the worst that could happen? As my gym rent was covered for another 2–3 months, it wasn't the end of the world if they didn't want to pay the fees. Psychologically I could go into the consultations with a lot more confidence and know that if they tried to haggle, I could turn them away. In some respect, I was buying an element of financial freedom and it worked very well.

FINANCIAL PROGRESSIVE OVERLOAD

Everyone knows you must add weight to the bar to get bigger and stronger. It goes without saying that making small, manageable increases in load each week is a great way to progress in you're training. So why not do it with your finances?

Let's translate this to the weights room and look at things from a hypothetical strength training point of view. You can squat 160 kg for one and your goal is to increase this to 200 kg. This is a 20–25% increase. Writing down "I squat 200 kg" every day may be a good idea (trust me, I've done it), but it won't do much good if you're not acting appropriately as well. You need a well-planned, thought out, systematic process to achieve your goal. You need to think about weaknesses, loading parameters, and most importantly, getting out of your comfort zone. Adding more and more weight each week isn't always the smartest thing to do. Going 165, 170, 175 may work, but it isn't optimal. You need to assess your foundations and establish what your strong points are, where you're lacking, and where most of your income comes from. Let's look at an example of how you could increase your earning potential by 20% in six months. This is a 3.3% growth in revenue every four weeks.

. When I asked my Facebook group, "How much can a PT earn per month?" the most common answer was £4,000. Using this as a baseline, let's look at how someone could grow by 20% from £3,400 to £4,000. Say your current earnings are £3,400 a month. Your first job before anything else is to assess your business and lock in the foundations. If someone wanted to get a strong squat, I'd first advise them to practice their technique and ensure they squat really well. There's no point in adding bands and chains to a poor movement pattern. The financial equivalent to this is getting your existing clients on direct debits, lock in their times, and make them happy. One of the fundamental aspects of growing a PT business is retaining clients. So, 3.3% of £3,400 is £112.20. This could easily equate to one new online client per month whilst maintaining your current income. Therefore, your target for the next six months is to take on one new online client whilst retaining all of your current client base. This is a simple model but if you follow it, your income would increase by 20% in six months. It seems so much easier when you break things down and do the maths. Now let's say you charge £35 an hour. You sign up a new client on a direct debit training twice a week. This is £280 extra income a month (roughly an 8% growth). Now you are technically ahead of your target by eight weeks. Your job now is purely to focus on client satisfaction. Make sure that your current clients are so happy that they daren't lose you. They should all be getting results and if their lifestyle doesn't permit them to drop weight each week, they should at least have the best training experience with you possible.

What is the moral of this story? Growth may seem difficult, but it's not if you create a plan and cement your current business. Don't treat your business as just earning a living; treat it as a company with set financial targets, goals, and incentives. The only difference is that you're not answering to anyone but yourself. Achieving your financial goals becomes infinitely easier if you can see the path to take you there. Calculate your numbers, look at the products you have to offer, and then write sales goals for that month. For example, one new one-to-one client training twice per week, one new online client, zero clients leaving.

Rinse and repeat this process for years on end and you'll eventually find your income doubling or even tripling. There is no magical formula or sales tools. Your business will improve when you dissociate yourself from the personal aspect of rejection and focus on hitting sales targets that are clear and precise. This doesn't take any emphasis away from your passion for the industry. It gives you a much better chance at creating a service and brand that can help you improve the lives of others. Businesses don't grow by accident. Progressively overload your income by knowing exactly what you need to do.

A NEEDS ANALYSIS OF PERSONAL TRAINING

Do you lack confidence in selling sessions because you're unsure whether people actually need you or not? I used to think I was bothering people more than helping them in the gym. Over the years my mindset has dramatically changed. I genuinely believe that absolutely everyone could benefit from a having a personal trainer. Let's have a look at why.

When I worked in a commercial gym, as far as I was aware it had around 7,000 members. A large portion of them would rarely use the gym. Commercial gyms aren't daft; they know that it's good for business to have dormant members. It's like a passive stream of income. These are the people who sign up and pay for a monthly membership, yet never actually use the gym at all. You'd be amazed at how many people do this. Out of the 7,000 active members, I'd estimate about 2,000 use the gym regularly. Based on these numbers, if I were to walk into a commercial gym today, there would be maybe 1,500 people who use the gym between open and close. I would confidently say that 90% of these people don't actually know what they're doing. Most people who go to gyms don't know anything about programme design, exercise selection, exercise execution, tempo, rest periods, or intensity. It's a completely foreign concept to them. They'll use the machines and do three sets of 10–20 depending on whether they like the exercise. These people would benefit a great deal from having someone teach them how to do the exercises, correct their technique, ensure they're working the right muscle, and monitor how hard they're working. If 90% of people in the gym need a trainer to show them how to train, this leaves 10% who are competent at training. Out of the 10% (roughly 150 people), how many of them do you think know exactly what to eat, at what time, in what amounts to fit their goals? How many of them could write a well thought out, scientifically sound macro plan that accounts for every gram? How many of them do you think would know how to change the plan and increase/decrease food amounts based on what they're trying to achieve. I'd say 20%, max. This leaves us with thirty people. Out of these, how many do you think would turn up, no matter what, come rain or shine, and train to their absolute maximum every single session? How many would make sure they milk every single rep for all that it's worth, squeezing the muscle under tension intently, chasing the pain of lactic acid instead of shying away from it? By now we're left with the hardcore lot, but I'd say 50% of these people at best. This leaves us with fifteen. Out of a membership base of 7,000, fifteen people don't need a personal trainer. That's 0.2% for the statistically inclined.

Of course, this is all a hypothesis. My point, however, is that having a good personal trainer is a necessity. In my experience, you seldom come across anyone in the gym who wouldn't benefit from having someone monitor their technique, intensity of training, nutrition, and lifestyle. In fact, I know that I'd hugely benefit from this. There are blurred lines when it comes to health and fitness. If you took a supercar around a racetrack or went jumping out of an airplane, it's likely they'd spend a lot of time going through safety precautions and how to do things properly. People completely overlook this aspect of the gym because many assume they know what they're doing. I'm more than happy to admit I did the same when I started lifting weights in my youth. It's an ego thing. And what about those who don't go to the gym? What about the people who want to get in shape but don't know where to start? They have insecurities, apprehension, and are confused about what they should be doing and what they should be eating. How invaluable would it be to them to have someone who will assess their habits, keep them accountable, give them dietary advice, and train them in a manner that isn't detrimental to their joints? Most people view personal trainers as a nice thing to have if you're affluent. They're an accessory, something that you invest in if you have lots of disposable income.

Although this is a common belief, I disagree. A personal trainer who sorts out your nutrition will improve the quality of your thinking. You'll be more productive and more efficient. I've had loads of my clients tell me they have tons more energy since starting training. When businesspeople have more energy and are more productive, they make more money. The return they see in their profits will make you an asset, not a disposable friend who escorts you around the gym. A personal trainer who understands the importance of tracking variables will improve your health markers. They'll be able to lower morning blood sugar, reduce blood pressure, improve mobility, and increase stability. This will reduce the likelihood of sick days or having to pay for surgeries in the future. If you are self-employed, taking a sick day is extremely costly. Therefore, minimising them is at the best of your interests. A personal trainer who is intent on self-development, who reads, writes, and educates themselves can install this mindset in their clients as well. This will increase their own sense of wellbeing and confidence, which will carry over into their work. If you dedicate yourself to becoming the best trainer you can possibly be, you go from being a **want to** have to being a **must** have.

The reality is, pretty much everyone needs your services, but whether they use them or not depends on how well you communicate your value. The better you get, the more in demand you will become. It's as simple as that. You'll be amazed at how many people can afford a decently priced PT. They just haven't invested yet because they haven't understood the value you can bring. Once you get through to someone, their perception of how you can help them will change.

We've established the value of having a personal trainer, now let's discuss the financial logistics of affording one. Pricing will be the biggest resistance you face from most people who do a consultation with you. They like the thought of having a PT, but they then need to justify the investment to themselves, family, and friends.

Do you think Ferrari salesmen struggle to sell their cars due to price? It's a serious question. Do you think people come in to the show room, take the car out for a test drive, but then say, "I'm sorry, it's a little out of my price range." I'm sure it's happened once or twice, but it won't be a common occurrence. If you're looking to buy a Ferrari, you need to have a certain amount of income. If the average Ferrari costs £100,000, it's safe to say you'd need to be a millionaire to purchase the car. But why is this? Everything that people spend their money on is proportional to their earnings. If I said to you, would you be happy with earning £150,000 a year? You'd probably say yes. It's a fantastic wage to be on. However, if a person earning this amount of money went out and bought a £100,000 car, they'd have just spent 66% of their annual income on one purchase. They'll have gone from being on a great wage to having to live off a relatively small amount of money given that their other expenses are probably pretty high. The point is that spending is all relative to your income. Your necessities hold primary importance, with all the bells and whistles being added on top. This is just the practicality of life.

The average wage in the UK for someone working full time is around £30,000 a year. This works out at £2,500 a month. If the average mortgage is paying back £750 a month, 30% of someone's monthly income goes on paying for where they live. Having a place to live is pretty important, so 30% of your income going on this isn't really too bad of a trade-off. But what else do people spend their money on? Car, food, petrol, phone bills, clothes? Well, the answer is, it depends. The percentage of which people spend their money on something will be dictated by what level of importance they put on that factor. Someone who goes out a lot and likes to wear nice things may spend 10–20% of their income on shopping per month. It's all down to what means the most to that person. How much they spend comes down to their own common sense and responsibility.

Where does personal training fit in? If we say that a personal training session is £30 an hour in a place where the average income is £30,000 per annum, seeing a trainer twice per week would cost you £240 per month. This fits in at 9.6% of monthly income. That's pretty affordable if you ask me. What can be deducted from these figures? I'd say that in general people will be happy to part with 10% of their monthly income on a luxury service. This being said, we've already established that if you cover training, nutrition, stress management, and habit formation with a client, that the 10% they invest in you is starting to look like money well spent.

Here we have established two clear notions. The first is that with perception of value comes an increase in delegation of monthly spends in that area. The second is that the more someone earns, the more they can spend on you. It may sound so obvious but when you break it down it provides valuable information for a business model. Your goal as a business should be to increase the value you provide. As well as this, you must target a clientele who can afford the rates you wish to charge. You don't *have* to do this, but if you want your hourly rate to reflect the effort you put into your education and services, demographics becomes a big thing. If we use the rule of 10%, what happens when you have a client who brings in £25,000 a month? Even if they were to spend 5% of their monthly income on you, this would mean over £100 a session if they were doing three sessions a week. It's important to know that even though we get hung up on hourly rate, it is literally just a drop in the ocean for some people. An hourly rate can even become arbitrary if you know how to communicate. Once you are at a point where you're so confident in your ability to get results with people, you could negotiate fees that don't even consider what you charge per hour.

Goal: Lose 20 kg
Time Frame: 24 Weeks
Conditions: Diet plan, supplement plan, cardio plan, three one-to-one sessions per week
Evaluated Cost: £5,000

Imagine selling PT blocks like that?

I know what you're thinking. I make it sound too easy when it's written down like that. You know what? I agree. If I had read this 7–8 years ago I would have laughed and said, "Yeah right." However, consider this: £5,000/6 = £833 a month. If this was 10% of someone's earnings, it means their annual income would need to be £100,000 a year. Is this an uncommon wage? Perhaps, but I'm sure there are many doctors, dentists, lawyers, and business owners who bring in this figure a year. They may even have had to sacrifice their health and undergo a lot of stress to get to where they are professionally. If someone offered to dramatically improve your health for a minor fraction of your annual income, would you take it? This is the biggest problem with personal training: we as trainers don't value the impact we can have on people. A well skilled, passionate, professional trainer is worth their weight in gold. Some people spend tens of thousands of pounds on one-week holidays, only to come back in worse shape than when they left. You're offering them a chance to buy their health back over a six-month period for what is, in retrospect, a pretty reasonable price.

Personal trainers are the world's first line of defence against many muscular skeletal and health issues. Don't believe me? What do most people ask their personal trainer about? They ask about how to move and what to eat. What are two of the biggest factors that contribute to injuries and our overall wellbeing? Our quality of movement and the quality of our diet. People take what their local PT or fitness professional say as the gospel (especially if you happen to be in good shape yourself). Therefore, a trainer can have a monumental impact on someone's belief system when it comes to nutrition and training. With great power comes great responsibility. People **do** need PTs and they **can** afford them. It all boils down to how well that PT presents themselves and shows value.

What now? Do we all change our pricing structure to blocks of £5,000? Do we increase our fees to £100 an hour? Obviously not. Just like weight training, it's about patient, progressive overload over time. You need to periodise a plan so that in two, three, or even five years' time, you are in a position where things are on your terms. You need to earn this right; you need to plan, and you need to be in it for the long game. Personal training can be an extremely lucrative career, but only for the ones who are willing to put the work in and be able to demonstrate value. If this is something you're passionate about, I want to make sure you achieve it.

BUILDING YOUR CLIENT BASE

It's fine talking about sales, but it doesn't bode well if you don't actually have anyone to sell to. Lead generation is an incredibly important aspect of personal training. It's all about numbers, energy, and the biggest thing of all, getting out of your comfort zone. If you're new to the industry, I recommend training as many different people as you can. Train people of different ages, abilities, backgrounds, and goals. It will build character. Later, specification is key to building a niche business that generates its own leads. Here are five things to consider for creating your ideal client.

1. Have a niche

It's important that you don't advertise yourself as a jack of all trades. Once you've identified the area you'd like to specialise in, make sure people are aware of it. As soon as you're known as the person to see about X or Y in your gym, you've nailed it, especially if there is a demand for this commodity. This really should only be one or two things. Would you go to KFC for a doughnut? Probably not, it's not something they're known for specialising in. Sure, they may sell doughnuts in some format, but I doubt they'll be as good as Krispy Kreme. Become known for being very good in one area. Make it the one you enjoy the most. As your career develops as a PT, you want to ensure that you're going in the right direction. When you start in the industry, it's difficult to be so selective straight away. You end up taking on people who have different needs and goals because you just want to get busy. Being busy in the early days is good, and I'd never recommend otherwise. However, the more advanced you get, the opposite is true. You want to get good at helping more specific demographics and know the bespoke problems they may have. When I worked in a commercial gym, I was obsessed with strength and conditioning. I studied textbooks religiously and read up as much as I possibly could on elite level performance. The problem was that my clients were all in their late thirties to forties, trained once or twice a week at best, didn't have the proper mechanics to execute compound movements correctly, and weren't particularly motivated to achieve their goals. My interest didn't match my demographic and I was getting frustrated. Now that my niche is more specific, most people who come to see me are looking to correct a movement pattern. My advice is to have a certain level of consistency in your posts on social media and what you talk about. Don't have content ADHD and go from Olympic lifting technique to pre- and post-natal training to gut health analysis. Just post about one topic 90% of the time and make sure it's the one that you enjoy the most. Imagine people coming to work with you and all they want to go through is an area you love and have expertise in. How good would that be?

2.   Honesty

Lay your cards on the table as early as possible, be it during the initial messaging, phone call, or consultation. Tell them what to expect, what they'll need to do, and what happens when they're not compliant. Use the bad experiences you have had and explain this to potential clients. You need to explain that their lack of compliance will be to their detriment and that you purely want them to get the most for their investment. It may look something like this.

Trainer: "I appreciate that your lifestyle can be hectic. However, I will require you to send a check-in with information for me so I can make any dietary or training adjustments. This is so you get the most out of my services and knowledge. In the event you forget to check in, I'll send an email to prompt you. This is a gentle reminder so that you know to send it. This does, however, have a three-strike rule. If a check-in is missed more than three times during a training phase, I won't be sending reminders again."

I know that sounds abrupt, but it works. You could re-word it to sound a bit less formal but it goes a long way with people to know where they stand. Worst case scenario, they'll realise you're not willing to take their money and leave them to it. It shows them that you care.

Second, be brutally honest with them at the start of the training journey. If someone who is 100kg and 30% body fat wants to look like a Men's Health cover model in twelve weeks, it is your job to explain that that simply isn't possible in a safe manner. Yes, it's possible for them to lose 20–25kg in that time, but the pursuit of muscle and fat loss is a tricky one. Tell people what they need to do, what to expect, and about the hunger, lifestyle changes, and discipline it will require. Your methods work, I know that and you know that. The only thing stopping someone from getting a result is how they apply themselves. You need to make sure they understand this during the consultation so you don't need to explain it down the line when it might be too late.

3.   Pass off the hagglers

The second someone starts to haggle with you, alarm bells should go off. It is critical that you do not break when someone tries to get a deal out of you. Whether it be in person or online, if you succumb to someone who manages to knock your price down, it can be extremely detrimental to your business.

Say you charge £35 an hour and £350 for a block of ten. You're doing a consultation and a person says, "Can you do it for £300?" It's near the end of the month, rent is due, and in a moment of weakness you agree. There are several reasons you are better off not taking the money. First, this person will now expect it for this price for the rest of the time they are training with you. If you say later that it's £350, now there is nothing to stop them from saying, "How come? Why were you able to do it for £300 in the first place?" Remember, people can be blunt and will take advantage of young naive trainers who aren't savvy with money, especially some business owners who are experienced in sales interactions. This isn't me being negative, it's just speaking from experience.

Second, if they refer a friend, they'll expect it for the same price. You'll risk the referral saying, "How come it's more for me?" It's hard to up your prices for someone who's friends with an existing client. It looks like you're inconsistent with your prices and this is a big sign of weakness in business.

Third, what do you do when you invest in a course or improve your services that means you now warrant increasing your rates? You'd be increasing this person's hourly rate to what you wanted to charge them in the first place. This is dumb.

Finally, what about existing clients? We all have at least one of those clients who is as good as gold, pays you on time, never argues about your rate, sings your praises, and has been with you for years. If they're paying £35 an hour and then you give a new customer a deal for £30, how do you think they'll feel? You may even risk losing them.

Hagglers are extremely bad for business. Not only for the reasons above but because they stand for one incredibly negative thing. Every time you train them, you are reminding yourself that you have been devalued. You are reminding yourself that you can easily be broken down and manipulated under pressure. These people make you feel bad about yourself. The worse thing is, they're almost always the people who don't get results.

If someone doesn't see value in you, then they won't take what you say seriously. They won't be compliant and they'll just see you as another expense they managed to trim. Them haggling you down is a way for them to feel better about themselves. What's worse is that they're likely to blame you when they don't get results. Trust me when I say this: sometimes you're much better off without the money. It's tough, but it will be worth it in the long run.

Remember, you have the power, not them. They need your services, but you don't need their money. What they pay you is simply an exchange for the excellent services you provide. Don't have an emotional attachment to it. Your price is your price, end of story. If people don't want to pay it, be polite, be professional, and advise them on the most suitable trainer you could recommend within their budget.

Hagglers are toxic. Never take them on.

4. Lay the rules early

When you take someone on as a client, you enter two relationships: how you interact as people and how you do business with each other. The personal relationship is the banter you have and the rapport you build. The business relationship is how you deal with exchanging money, how you deal with cancellations, and drawing the line where you both stand as friends. That's the biggest issue with personal training, which in my opinion is bespoke to the field. When you end up spending time with someone, you'll eventually get familiar with them and end up becoming friends. This has its positives and negatives.

Becoming a "rent-a-friend" is a risky situation for you and your business. It has happened to me before where I felt like I was spending most of the session talking rather than working hard. This isn't good for you, it isn't good for your client, and it certainly isn't good for the people watching around the gym.

This doesn't mean you can't be friendly. People will stay with you because of the relationship you build with them. However, you must start how you mean to go on.

- Explain in the first consultation that all cancellations without twenty-four hours' notice are charged.
- Keep texting at the weekend to a minimum and try not to discuss any other topic other than health and nutrition with your client.
- Don't take freebies, use holiday homes, or take liberties from affluent clients, even if they can afford it.
- Always have a stopwatch on you in your session so that you can time rest intervals. This is so you don't spend five minutes in between sets of bicep curls talking about football results.

When you see clients 3–4 times a week, it's easy to become friends with them. That then gives them the temptation for "mate's rates" or to become slack with training. For people to get results, they need to see you as an authority figure, not a friend.

You need to make sure there are no blurred lines with your client relationships. If you use their holiday home at the weekend, you definitely won't be able to charge if they let you down last minute. The gratification you get from accepting a gift that you think you'll enjoy is actually a detriment to your business. In their eyes, your business should be doing so well that they don't need to give you anything for free. You're a businessperson, so act like one.

Successful businesspeople who invest in your services are where they are for a reason. They'll be good at figuring people out, good at business transactions, and know how to handle people. The firmer and more professional you are, the more they'll respect your time

5. Create a package that suits you, not them

When I worked in a commercial gym, they sold packs of three or ten sessions. I presumed they did this so it seemed more affordable for the members who were already paying an extortionate amount for the club and leisure facilities. The thing is, ten sessions is as arbitrary as ten reps. As we know, there is nothing special about ten reps during a set, and the same goes for sessions.

The fact of the matter is, ten sessions isn't a lot. People need high frequency personal training because they simply aren't knowledgeable or skilled enough to train themselves as well as you'd be able to train them. You have skills they require—don't ever forget that. If you charge £40 an hour and someone is seeing you once a week, my advice is to say you'll train them three times a week for £30. Yes, you may have reduced hourly rate by £10, but you'll have more than doubled the weekly spend with you to £90. They feel like they're saving money but in reality, they've spent more. You get more money, they get more training, and everyone's a winner.

What if you were to sell a block of thirty-six sessions? This is three per week for twelve weeks. Remember, people can't buy something that doesn't exist. The only reason someone hasn't bought a large block of sessions from you is because you don't have it available to buy. Once it's there, it's an option. Ask yourself, "What terms would I like?" If you want to train people once per week, then offer them once per week. If you don't think once a week training works, then don't offer it. Remember, you're the professional and you know what works. If 2–3 times a week training minimum works, then this is the only thing you should offer.

Attracting new clients is one of the most important aspects of growth. It's something that I struggled with for years and didn't know where to start. A lot of it boiled down to lack of self-confidence and fear of rejection. Some trainers are good at creating and converting leads; others may be good client retention and keeping people happy. A lot of it depends on your personality type and background. When working in a commercial gym, I was taught that the best way to generate leads was to give away a taster session. We'd be prompted to walk the gym floor, approach people whilst they were training, and offer them a free one-to-one PT session. Maybe I'm not the best at chatting up random people in the gym, but I'd say the amount of gym goers who were responsive to this type of treatment was around 20%. Most people just wanted to be left alone and crack on with their own thing. Out of the 20% who spoke to you, most would be polite but realise your motives and then make up some excuse as to why they couldn't book in. Some people do the opposite and smell the opportunity for a freebie. I think this is important to know for trainers who are new to the industry so they don't take it personally. The person may have loved the session you did with them. They may have thought you're a brilliant trainer. However, some people just book in purely because they can and have no intention of buying anything.

Let's look at this from a different angle. People are more likely to buy when the product on offer serves a purpose or solves a problem. Take the iPhone for example. The technology to develop it probably cost billions, but the object itself probably doesn't cost that much to make. Therefore, you're not paying for the value of the phone, you're paying for the investment in technology to make sure your phone does everything you want it to do. See where I'm going with this? The reason people are happy to part with hundreds, if not thousands of pounds for a phone is because it does a lot of things very well. Now, let's imagine that the iPhone hadn't been released yet and Apple were doing a massive marketing campaign to get people interested in purchasing them. Which one do you think would be the most successful?

Campaign 1:
Would you find it more convenient if all your utilities were wrapped up in to one small, easy to store and manoeuvre device?
Do you want access to all your favourite TV shows, websites, social media outlets and music in the palm of your hand?
Would you find it easier to be able to do online shopping, banking, transactions and accounts all from a light, portable handheld device?
We have the solution for you. Introducing, the iPhone.

This marketing campaign speaks to the reader by identifying a problem and showing a solution. It grabs their interest, and now it is down to them to make the inquiry in to how much it costs. When it comes to a business transaction, you always want the potential client to ask you for the price rather than for you to tell them. If they do this, it shows that buying the product is something they're considering.

Now let's look at Campaign 2. This isn't a media or written campaign, its people standing around a busy shopping centre with a big stand that says iPhone on it (bearing in mind that hypothetically no one knows what an iPhone is).

Person goes up to passer by
"Excuse me, Sir, would you like to try out our new handheld device? It can link to the internet, call people, do banking…"
Man walks away slightly disgruntled that he's been interrupted

People generally don't like being stopped whilst they're doing things. Think about your own experience when shopping. What do you do when you clock someone who's going to try to stop you and sell car insurance or Sky TV in a shopping mall? You usually put your head down and walk the other way. This is especially true if you have something important to do and need to get it done quickly.

Now, let's say someone does stop and have a look at the iPhone. They like what they see and think it's a great little product. You've won them over but when you explain it costs £500, they're outraged and hastily make an excuse as to why they need to get going. Here's the thing: it's not that this person didn't think the iPhone wasn't worth that, it's just that they weren't expecting to part with such a large amount of money from a fleeting transaction. Imagine what would happen if all it took was someone to stop you in the street and talk to you and you'd part with hundreds of pounds each time. You'd be broke very quickly.

To gain people's attention for personal training, you need to do two things: provide the solution to a problem they have and make sure that they're in the market. It would be pretty dumb for an estate agent to send a load of fliers to a brand-new housing estate where every single person on there has just moved house. Think about the people you are selling to. Your goal should be to engage with them and get them to make the first move. Wear a t-shirt that says Personal Training on it, so eventually they'll ask, "Do you offer PT?" This is your opportunity to say, "Yes, I certainly do. Would you like to book in for an assessment session?" No matter what gym you're in, be it commercial or an independent facility, you must treat every person in there as if they're your client. Why? Because they could be. You don't know how long someone may be assessing or saving to work with you. It's critical that you speak to everyone—and I do mean everyone—about their goals, training, and lifestyle. Do not give anyone the opportunity to say, "I've never spoken to that PT because they don't seem approachable." Just talk, be friendly, and offer as much advice as you can without letting people take liberties.

If someone asked me what my niche is, I'd definitely say movement assessments. It doesn't have the best ring to it, but it interests me the most. I've fallen into this niche due to the amount of injuries I've had. I've hurt myself several times lifting weights and want to make sure that it never happens again. The funny thing is, the more balanced and less injury prone you are, the more you'll be able to lift as well. It works both ways.

Another reason for wanting to learn more about correctional exercise is that I've noticed such a large volume of people in commercial and independent gyms do things wrong. You can see that their form is off and their mobility is poor, and you can't help but think, "I'm sure this will be doing more damage than good." I've always wanted to get people the best results possible. This is not necessarily just body composition (as this depends a lot on psychology and lifestyle circumstances), but more so being strong and pain free—maximising your mechanics, if you will. What has this got to do with generating leads? I'll explain later. First, I need to explain how to maximise giving your time away and why.

If you're going to give away a free session, there are certain things I recommend doing beforehand with the potential client to avoid disappointment. You don't want to make things seem like a hard sell, but you don't want to get fobbed off at the end of the session. The last thing you want is someone to say, "Okay, thanks mate" and walk off. It can happen and makes you feel stupid.

The first thing I recommend is to explain to the potential client the goal of the session. This could be something along these lines:

"Today is going to be a little insight into what we would do in a typical one-to-one session. If you feel like training would benefit you, you can purchase more sessions for the cost of X for Y."

I recommend doing this from the start because now you have at least desensitised them to the investment of training. They know they're with you free of charge for the next hour but will be constantly thinking, "Is this going to be worth the money?" Here comes your time to shine. What I wouldn't do in any taster session is try to do anything fancy. Complicating things and trying to design the most bespoke, unique session in the world doesn't make you a great coach; being great at coaching makes you a great coach. If you beast a client with the most brutal circuit session ever, they'll associate you with pushing them to their limit. This is good, but a spin or aerobics class can do this, and they are included in their membership. You need to show them a level of value that they couldn't replicate.

I ask the person at the beginning of the session what they usually do in the gym. I want to know which exercises they perform, why they do them, and how long they've been doing it for. In my opinion, there is absolutely nothing more powerful than taking them through their own workout while showing them how much better it could be if you were there. Let's look at an example. It may sound cliché, but it has actually happened to me in a commercial gym.

Trainer: So, what exercises do you usually do in the gym?

Taster client: Bench press, then some pull ups, then some machines.

Trainer: Okay cool. Let's have a look at this exercise then.

Walk over to the bench press

Trainer: How much can you do on here?

Taster client: About 80kg for five reps.

Trainer: Cool, let's see it.

Man proceeds to put a 20 kg plate either side of the bar and do ten reps of the fastest eccentrics you've seen in your life. The first six are good, the seventh is a bit off, and the eighth to tenth reps are horrible grinders with elbows everywhere and hips humping the bar up to the top. You also notice that his chest isn't very big.

Trainer: So what's your goal here?

Taster client: I just want to fill in the upper portion of my chest as I feel it's lacking compared to the rest of my chest.

Trainer: Okay, let's try a different approach.

Now comes your time to demonstrate true value. Whilst training him, ask yourself if he could replicate this training technique and intensity without you there. Teach him about tempo, make him reduce the weight and learn about control, cue how to engage a muscle and stop him from cheating, add pauses, and help the bar up slightly. Then you need to make him feel like he's just done the hardest set of his entire life and only used 40 kg. This will be an eye opener for him.

After the bench press, you can explain that dumbbells may be more optimal for hypertrophy due to the greater range of movement. You can then use lighter weights again and torch his chest in a way he's never done before. In the hour slot, you only do 6–8 working sets, but the rest of the time is spent cueing, teaching, and educating him where he's gone wrong. Think of a taster session as a return in investment. Don't try to hammer someone; anyone can do that. You must show your value in a way that the potential client realises you're not just some person who hangs around the gym. If you think it's giving all your best info away for free, then don't worry, it's not. The person will only be able to retain about half the things you said to them. You can almost guarantee they won't be able to replicate the same intensity again and they'll always have questions. They'll also be likely to tell other gym goers about you: "I did a session with that trainer and wow, it was eye opening."

My point is, showing people where they've been going wrong is more valuable than showing them something new. Investing is all about finding something that solves your problems and not necessarily novelty. Personal trainers shouldn't be entertainers; they are there to give gym goers the best possible session and remove the thinking for them. That's essentially why anyone subsidises anything: to make their life easier by bringing in an expert in that field.

To grow, you have to get out of your comfort zone, accept that failure is a part of growth, and understand that rejection is just a way of making yourself stronger.

Now, imagine if you'd done the same session with that potential client but with 4–5 people instead. Imagine how good you'd look being in the weights area, tutoring some gym goers, and torturing some poor soul with 40 kg on the bar. How would this approach seem to you? You're saving time, increasing your potential buying audience, and improving your image around the gym. Rather than calling this type of thing a taster (which is free and means it's devalued), how about something like Bench Press Workshop. This is where you'll teach a client some basic tips (to you) on how they can improve their pressing skills. You could create a poster and put it in the free weights area. Remember, ask the questions they'll be asking themselves.

Bench Press Workshop - Every Monday 6:00-6:30pm

Do you struggle to feel your chest whilst pressing?
Have you plateaued in the bench and don't know why?
Would you like to know ways of getting both big and strong in the bench press?
The Bench Press Workshop will teach you all of this. Available this Monday at 6:00, limited to five people.

You can do this for any area: running workshop, core workshop, deadlift workshop, and so forth. The most important thing is to ask questions that people will want answered. Remember that a lot of people will be shy to ask questions, and the more you're willing to help, the more relationships you'll build. From a lead generation perspective, your goal is to put yourself in a position where people can see what you have to offer. You can do this through interactions on the gym floor and running regular workshops showcasing your knowledge. Always ask yourself, how can I demonstrate value and make myself a necessity, not a nicety?

I have had some people say that workshops like this shouldn't be free. If you believe this too, charge a fee for these presentations. The only issue in commercial gyms may be payment, as the company will not like you taking cash in hand on the gym floor. Another complication is that if they pay via reception, how do you receive the money? I'm not saying not to charge, I'm just saying you might encounter some complications. If you work in an independent facility and feel like these workshops are worth charging for, be my guest.

WALKING THE GYM FLOOR

Floor walking is one of the most difficult aspects of working in a commercial gym. If you're new to personal training and go to a job interview, it's likely that they'll ask you to walk around the gym floor and speak to 3–5 people. It can be terrifying, especially when you're new to the industry and are shy by nature. The first thing I want you to know is that if you find it daunting, you're not alone. Here's what I've learned in the trenches of walking the gym floor.

I'm sure a lot of coaches will wholeheartedly admit they don't relish having to do forced interactions. This being said, it is actually an important component of personal training that you'll will need to face and overcome. My view on the industry is quite simple. You need to be one of four things to be taken seriously or stand out: big, ripped, strong, and smart. If you tick at least two of the boxes, you may make the grade of "legit trainer" in most people's eyes. My point is that people are superficial and will judge without knowing you. If it's not glaringly obvious that you might offer them something of value, they may not be so willing to give you their time. The guy who's jacked and in great shape will always get asked more questions than any other trainers regardless of knowledge, skill set, or qualifications. If you feel you don't fall into any of the four categories just yet, don't worry; it's still the early stages of your career and this is totally acceptable. As you proceed, work hard to get to a decent standard in a certain discipline, be it strength sports, physique training, or endurance running. Have something that makes you a specialist in one area.

When I worked in a commercial gym, I was very much in to powerlifting. I wasn't big or particularly ripped but I became a little bit more credible to the guys in the weights section for being able to squat and deadlift over 180kg. I had extremely poor technique, but it was the blind leading the blind and they just recognised weight, not form. I started many a conversation in the weight area just from people coming over and stating the obvious: "That's a lot of weight you've got on there." Now, I'll be the first to admit I was doing things wrong, but it opened doors and helped me interact with people who would otherwise be difficult to engage. If you want to find it easier and less intimidating to talk to people on the gym floor, make it your objective to break down their superficial judging by relentlessly working on getting really big, strong, ripped, or smart. If you do this, your business will sell itself.

If you train hard and intelligently, people will eventually approach you. They'll ask why you're adding bands to things; they'll be intrigued by the colourful drink you're sipping; they'll want to know more about what you're doing—especially if they can see you're making progress each week. Remember, you don't have to be the biggest or strongest, but people will want to talk to you if you're getting bigger and stronger. The guys doing horribly rounded back deadlifts and quarter range bench press and squats will be watching. You don't have to approach them, but when they see your weights and muscle bellies both increasing, whilst doing everything with perfect form, they'll eventually approach you. Trust me. Let's run through a little scenario.

You've just qualified as a PT and start working at a new gym. You've been training about three years and your goal is to put on as much muscle as you can. Being new to the game, your confidence in approaching people is pretty low, so you're just getting to terms with walking the gym floor. On your first shift in the gym, you find the free weights section is an absolute free for all, filled with a sea of grunting apes, none of them doing anything correctly and all of them leaving their dumbbells everywhere. Your first interaction with them is an intimidating one. No one makes eye contact with you and the person you try to smile at immediately turns away.

You decide to train at 5:00pm one evening. You perform five reps of perfectly executed deadlifts with a 4-0-1-0 tempo. On your last set, you notice a two lads watching the lift. You think nothing of it and carry on. As you want to get your name out there, you set up a stand with a sign that says "free core stability workshop" on a table by the door. It has a tagline:

> *Always feel your lower back when lifting?*
> *Do you regularly have lower back pain whilst sitting at your desk?*
> *Want to know simple yet effective ways to manage and overcome this?*
>
> *Free to all members between 5:00-5:30pm this Monday*

It doesn't get much interaction, but you leave it there. One day, you're doing your usual deadlift session, this time with 10 kg more than the last rotation, and notice the same guy from a few weeks ago watching your set. You finish your last rep and go to fill up your water bottle, and as you do, he seems to be hovering around the water fountain.

"You deadlifting today?"

Now, both of you know that you are, but this is just his way of breaking the ice. You nod as you're getting your breath back and filling up your water bottle.

"I used to deadlift all the time. My PB is 260 kg," he says.

"Oh nice, that's a good lift," you reply.

"Its proper hard though, isn't it? I had to stop because I messed up my back."

BINGO!

Remember that most people in the gym will have a niggle/injury that is holding them back. They don't want to ask the trainer for help as their ego will tell them not to. Either that or they'll worry about being sold something. In their head, they know what they're doing. I'm telling you now: no one in the gym really has a clue what they're doing. Think about it. His training education has more than likely come from magazines and social media. He won't understand anatomy, spinal mechanics, periodisation, or programme design. You do. This is the difference. All people require help, they just need to see how you can help them. If they can't see this, they'll never look to ask for help. You can now refer him to your workshop, which will explain simple ways he can improve his lower back health. Even if he's the only one who turns up to your workshop, you'll be creating a relationship with someone at the gym, which dramatically increases your value. Even if he can't afford one-to-one PT, your online services may be perfect for him.

We've spoken about how people like to be sold to and then discussed the importance of demonstrating value. Now I'm going to go through how you can develop a system that will make your taster sessions efficient and informative, but also an excellent way in which you can improve your knowledge. First, this isn't going to be some "teach you how to sell and convert" type of thing—far from it. It's going to be a simple explanation of to how you can design a taster session that you can do with every new inquiry. It's what I did many moons ago and is 100% what I would do if I were to go back to working in a commercial gym or wanted to increase my client base anywhere.

Instead of showing people how you'd train them, learn how to thoroughly screen people for movement discrepancies and mobility/stability issues. In my opinion, this is a superior way of spending time with people. Personal training is competitive. People type cast trainers and think we're just gym rats who eat protein and do bicep curls. It's a sad but true reality. It's important that you disarm a punter, show them that you have their best interests in mind, and demonstrate how you can help them. Most of the people you speak to will say things like:

"I want to get a bit bigger, but not too big."
"I'd just like to tone a bit and lose a bit of weight."
"I'd like to feel a little healthier."

Phrases like that are just things you'll have to get accustomed to when doing consults. You'll hear them time and time again. One of the most important questions I think you can ask in a consultation is, "Do you have any injuries?" This will usually spark a response of bad back, bad knees, bad shoulder, bad neck, and so on. It's safe to say that 9/10 people carry some sort of niggle with them most of the time and have no idea how to get rid of it. Enter the personal trainer.

I think of personal training as a double-edged sword. It's your chance to make someone stronger and injury free, or an opportunity to make them even worse. Most people in the gym are doing exercises they probably shouldn't be doing. Say someone comes to you with a bad knee. They've had a bad knee for years and it's gotten to the point where they now walk around with a 5/10 pain in their knee all the time. You're not a doctor but some simple screening tests could tell you a lot about what's going on. Instead of training them during a taster, you do a movement screening where you look at ROM in all the major joints. You see that the ankle on the problematic side has poor mobility and restricted external rotation of the hip. When you ask them if they do anything to strengthen the knee, they say, "I can't do squats anymore as it hurts too much, so I do leg extensions instead."

The fact that this person's pain may be stemming from lack of ankle and hip mobility and stability is completely alien to them. They wouldn't even think that the cause of the problem could be coming from somewhere else, and why would they? It's not their job. Do you ever take your car to a mechanic and know exactly what's going on with it already? This little bit of information you provide them could dramatically help them improve their standard of living. This is invaluable. Consider what you would rather someone say about you after a session: "That PT absolutely annihilated me. I thought I was going to die. I can barely walk now," or, "Wow, that PT really knows his stuff. He explained to me why my knee pain might not actually be my knee, it may be coming from my ankles and hip."

Screening sessions are an amazing way to learn about how the body moves. The problem with the PT industry is that we learn the best exercises for the hypothetical ideal structure of the body, so for example, a chest fly is the best way to stimulate the pec. This doesn't take into account having rounded shoulders, a shoulder impingement, short biceps, or weak stabilisers. All these factors play a part in exercise selection and its effectiveness. The best way for you to learn how to overcome these issues is to experience it in the field and decipher ways of overcoming the problem yourself. It's the ten thousand-hour rule of mastery. The more people you see, the more things will make sense to you, the better you will become at finding a solution.

Screening hundreds—yes, hundreds—of people will make you an infinitely better trainer. It is also the best way to learn functional anatomy and how certain joints are impacted by others. So how does this work well with a taster? Thorough screenings absolutely scream professionalism. They show that you care and show you are different to every other PT who just takes someone's money and then goes straight on to the gym floor. It will make you stand out. Furthermore, you have then already done your initial screening with them. Therefore, you already have the data you need to design their programme, which will save you time.

Finally, when it comes to the sell at the end of the taster, you can present the findings in a business-like manner. You can say, "This is what I found from the movement screening. The tightness in this muscle may be the reason you haven't been able to get rid of the pain in your knee. Whilst working together, I would be looking to help you improve this issue as well as providing diet information so that you can improve your nutritional knowledge. The goal over the next twelve weeks would be to lose a stone in weight and get your knee stronger and moving better." This system is much more efficient and effective because you get to learn. Even if your sign-up conversion rate isn't the best, people will respect you more if you can show them where their problems are and how you can help them. Be the type of trainer that improves the quality of a client's life, not makes it worse through improper selection of exercises and intensities.

LEAD GENERATION

This section is specifically for those who are new to the industry. It will explain things about sales, psychology, and working with the general population, all of which are important to understand. As I've said many times before, you need to be good at business and not just training people to survive in this industry. My goal is to help you to understand what I consider the universal laws of lead generation and sales.

Whenever I face an obstacle, I like to think I have a logical explanation and solution to the problem. Client won't stop talking? Buy a stopwatch to indicate rest times. Client is constantly late? Change their regular time to a later slot. Client can't lift with good technique? Change the exercise to accommodate their movement capabilities. Problem solving is an important part of growth and will help your business. One area that always presents a challenge is predicting forecasts from initial leads. I'm always tempted to predict the best-case scenario and over-estimate my earning potential. It's not a bad thing, but it can lead to frustration. One thing I've learned in business is to always be conservative with predictive figures and plan for the worst-case situation. Any business plan should account for making sure you at least break even.

Let's look at the concept of "hot leads" and "cold leads" and how, frustratingly, they can switch from one to the other at the drop of a hat. Hot leads and cold leads are an incredibly important component of business for several reasons. By the end of this chapter, I'd like you to understand why tracking them is essential, how you can convert a cold lead to a hot lead, and then in to active clients. First, let's go through what I mean by each term.

Hot Lead

You're working at a commercial gym and a potential member is being shown around the facility by the sales team. They're looking at the coaches' board and explain they'd like a PT to train them twice a week. You're called over, meet the inquirer, and get them booked in for a taster session next week. They sign up for the membership, come to your taster session, love what you have to offer, and say they're interested. This is what I would call a hot lead because:

- They have instigated the interest in training,
- They have already interacted with you in a positive way,
- You have trained them and they enjoyed the session,
- They are aware how much training costs,

Now, none of these actually mean the person is going to sign up. That, in some way, is still an arbitrary fact that works on the law of averages. What it does mean is that you have someone who has increased their likelihood of signing up with you by breaking down certain areas of resistance like the initial meeting, interaction style, or sales price. If someone is still showing active interest after knowing the price of something and trying the product, it means the chance of them buying is higher than someone who isn't familiar with those aspects. Hot leads are important because they increase the likelihood of you getting a bite. Imagine you are fishing in a pond and every hot lead you add to the equation is like putting a large, hungry fish in the water. As these increase, the chances of you catching a fish goes up.

Hot leads come from active interaction. They come from putting yourself out there, talking to people, and getting out of your comfort zone. If you're not an outgoing, extroverted person, you will need to embrace these qualities in order to improve lead generation. It's just the nature of the game. The main thing that makes someone a hot lead is breaking down resistance. They know price and they know you. It's now down to them to decide what to do next. The best thing to do with hot leads after an initial session is to exchange information and then have a call to action. People don't like to be put on the spot when it comes to buying, but if you're too flippant about a sale, they may get distracted by other things that are going on in their life. Give people a specific time that you will contact them to discuss their decision. For example: "If you would like start training you can purchase sessions by doing, X,Y,Z; however, I appreciate it if you need some time to think things through. I'll drop you a text in a couple days to see whether you'd like to book in." It is important you state that you will be contacting them and require a decision. Do not repeatedly message people, even if they seemed interested at the time. The more you message, the more you'll seem desperate for business. If they don't get back to you or respond to your call to action text, change them to a cold lead and move on.

Cold Lead

Cold leads are your long shots—the people who don't seem likely to buy and are more gaging interest to see what's what. They may inquire, but don't want to commit for fear of a hard sell. For example, you get chatting to someone on the gym floor and make small talk. You chat about sports, the weather, and get to know their name. After a couple of weeks of gaining familiarity, you ask them about their programme and what they do in the gym. You chat and it's pleasant and you consider to have built rapport them.

Despite this seeming like a good lead to pursue personal training, it's actually not. I'm not saying this person won't sign up, as there's every change they will. However, cast your mind back to the hot leads: instigated interest, positive interaction, enjoyed taster session, knows the price. If this person only ticks one box, then they're still in the cold category. Don't think about this from the vibe you get from the person. Look at it from black and white objective data. This isn't because this is an exact science, it's so you can then assess what you do with your time.

How do you get more clients? Put out deals? Increase social media posts? Walk the gym floor during peak times? Law of attraction? All of these are good points but don't really cut it in the business world. If I were your business coach as a PT, I would ask, "How many hot and cold leads do you have?" I wouldn't want estimates or off the top of the head accounts; I'd want numbers, names, and forecasts.

PT: "I need to get new clients."

"Can you tell me your current list of lead generation?"

PT: "I have four hot leads and three cold leads."

"What's the current state of the hot leads?"

PT: "One is currently away on holiday and said they'll get back to me once they return. One said they'll start at the beginning of next month and two haven't got back to me."

"Okay, great. Make sure you follow up those two by the end of next week and if you don't hear back from them, change them to cold leads and look to find new leads."

Ruthlessness when it comes to business is important. You can't dwell and take people's word for whether they will sign up. If you do, you'll procrastinate, wait with bated breath, and potentially lose income because you're not actively signing enough people up. I did it for years. You take people's word for it too much and think you're doing okay in your head, but weekly session delivery doesn't lie. If you're not as busy as you'd like to be, you need a systematic way of creating leads, converting leads, and sorting where to put your energy. Data is everything. If you know four hours per week on the gym floor generates ten leads and you convert two of them, you then have a formula on which to build. Formulas and correlations are essential for business growth.

People forget. They get family commitments. They may like the sound of having a PT but then realise the financial investment is too much. They get talked out of it by family and friends. They think they can do it themselves. They may even use another PT. Until they become an active, paying client, they are just a number. I'm not for a second saying you should view everyone you talk to just as money—far from it. However, do not dwell on people who may be wasting your time. Talk to them, help them, show them what you have to offer, and then contact them afterwards to see if they're interested. If they're not, move on.

Independent facilities

I think it was Tony Robbins who said that success leaves clues. Sometimes the best way of improving your business is to ask for help from those who've already achieved what you want to achieve. I'd love to say, "Here is a fool-proof plan for attracting clients," but I'm afraid I don't have a formula for that. Truth be told, I don't think anyone does. I think that all the "attract thirty new clients in thirty days" sales pitches are misleading. They may give you a script, but they don't account for your unique situation.

I was fortunate when I transitioned to a self-employed trainer. I'd been working as a PT for three years and had built up confidence and competency in the safety of a commercial gym. I say safety because although the money wasn't that great,

I didn't have to pay any rent at a time and my overheads were low. When I moved across to an independent facility, I took three clients with me. As I was local to the area, I trained a couple of my mum's friends just to get the ball rolling income wise. I'm talking one session a week charging £20 as a mate's rate. I was just looking to boost my income and get used to the life of the self-employed. Slowly but surely, my old clients from the commercial gym got back in touch. They asked where I was and came down to have a look at the gym. I sealed the deal by charging them £10 an hour less than what they were paying in the commercial gym (despite knowing they could pay it— everyone loves a bargain). I took classes at the gym when I could. This included circuit training sessions and strongman sessions on a Saturday. This got people used to my face and the type of training I liked to do. I also took an outdoor bootcamp class that my friend ran twice a week. This was growing nicely and so gave me an audience of around twenty people to talk to on a weekly basis.

Whilst I was at the commercial gym, I had struck up a referral system with the in-house health care practitioners. I sent all my clients to the physios and chiropractors there and they sent their patients to me. When I moved to the independent gym, I continued with this referral scheme with good success. I also posted on social media at least 3–4 times a week about nutrition or training.

When you go self-employed in a quieter, independent gym facility, lead generation becomes a whole different ball game. You have to work hard, tick boxes, and be proactive. If you don't, you'll lose momentum. Every day needs to count, and you have to make sure you:

- Post informative, useful content online 3–4 times per week,
- Make sure all the existing gym members know you and find you approachable,
- Do classes in and outside the gym for exposure and a way of getting people familiar with you,

- Have a referral scheme with a local health practitioner, and
- Provide the best possible service for your existing client base.

It is essential that you get your name out there even more than you would in a commercial gym. At commercial gyms, there's always the chance you may get someone who just signs up for PT with zero prompting. I remember being sat in the gym office in the commercial gym I worked at being frustrated and wondering how on earth to get new clients as a PT. Then, no word of a lie, this guy walks into the office and says, "Is this where you pay for PT?" I replied, "No, that's at reception, how come?" He said, "I'd like to buy some sessions. Do I do them with you?" However, it's highly unlikely this will happen in independent facilities.

I stuck to the above check list religiously during my first year as a self-employed PT. I put on free health seminars, gave introductory offers for the people in the bootcamps, and did free screenings for people in the strongman classes. I just put myself out there. One year on from going self-employed, I was averaging 35–40 sessions per week. This was the busiest I've ever been in my entire PT career. I wasn't charging exactly what I wanted, but I was busy and initially, that's all that matters. If ever in doubt, get busy first. Being busy will teach you the true value of time.

No one is going to do anything for you. If you're not proactive in earning money, no money will be earned. The time you spend aimlessly scrolling social media or watching Netflix is time you waste that could be spent working on your business. Leads will come naturally the more you put yourself out there. Even if it takes time, the harder you work, the luckier you get. One Sunday morning I got a call from the guy who owned our gym. He said that a group of lads who train in MMA want to come in for a group training session.

"I've priced them out of it," he said. "I've said it's £100 for the hour if they want to rent the gym. If they do turn up, we can go halves and I'll give you £50."

At the time, £50 for an hour's work was a massive amount of money for me. I was the second trainer he'd offered it to and as the first one didn't fancy it, I went along to do the session. I got there for 11:00 and there was no one in sight. I was expecting four hard as nails, Russian looking fighting machines to turn up any time. Five minutes went by, then ten, then fifteen. Still no one. Great, I'd come in to work on a Sunday for nothing. Eventually, at twenty-five past, four lads turned up who were far from athletes. They didn't really look like they trained, and I think one of them had been to a couple of MMA classes. They weren't exactly about to debut on the UFC. I did a basic strongman class with them. Prowler, sled, slam balls, sledgehammer, that type of thing. After twenty minutes they were all collapsed on the floor with a couple of them throwing up several times. As luck would have it, one of them was hooked. He asked how much it would be to train three times a week. I quoted him £30 a session and he booked in with two of his friends. They got each session for £10 and I was up £90 a week.

After about a month, the same lads brought some more of their friends down. I explained I couldn't do a session with six people, so they split into two groups. This worked out at £180 a week, £720 a month. They did this for well over a year. If you work it out, that's around eight and a half grand earned, just from going to work on a Sunday and putting yourself out there. Was I lucky? Yes, without a doubt. However, I believe that fortune favours the brave. Luck creates itself when you're willing to put the work in. If you're working in an independent facility and are concerned about getting new clients, create a check list of all the things you should be doing and do it without fail. Eventually you will be rewarded.

If you are like me, it's easy to get excited by new inquiries and jump the gun, thinking, "If they all sign up, this will be a good month." In this section, I'd like to explain what to do, what to put focus into, and look at a way to deal with your inquires in a systematic manner.

Before I begin though, I need to emphasise a critically important aspect of the personal training industry. This mindset is extremely hard to achieve but vital in the sense of longevity in the business. Simply put, you need to cut your emotional attachments to money. If you can do this, your business will improve.

Emotion is what makes us human. It's an evolutionary development that dictates our health, stature, and wellbeing. Being connected to your emotions, or at least in control of them, is a form of mastery of one's self. The more you can understand your emotions, the more you have control over your actions and therefore destiny. Why the profound statement? Well, our emotional attachment to money will always be a detriment to our ability to grow our business. If we fear money, we will neither be able to accept it or hold on to it. If we desire money, we don't have the ability to approach situations from a neutral perspective. Like the love-struck teenager who does absurd things for a high school crush, high levels of emotional attachment impact our ability to think logically.

Potential client after taster session: "Wow, I've never trained like that before. What availability do you have again?"

Trainer: "I can do Monday, Wednesday, Friday at 9am."

Potential client: "Perfect. I can drop the kids off at school, then head here before going into the office for 10:30am. How much did you say it is a month?"

Trainer: "£480 on direct debit."

Potential client: "Okay great. Send me your bank details and I'll get that sorted once I'm back from my holiday next week."

Sounds like a great interaction, right? The only thing is, a week later you don't hear anything back. You text them, no reply. You email, no reply. This hot lead goes completely quiet on you to the point where you start to give up completely. Three weeks and numerous texts and emails later, you call it quits.

How does this make you feel? Angry, sad, annoyed, hard done by? Yep, I've felt all of those. You almost feel betrayed, as if someone has promised you money then cruelly taken it away. It's not a nice aspect of personal training, but it is the reality. Even though it's incredibly difficult, you must approach everything as neutral in this situation. You must be stoic; you must be impervious to outcomes and steely in your business mindset. If someone doesn't sign up, so what? Move on, keep working hard, and keep to the formula. One of my best business mentors, Geoff Sober, once said, "Some will, some won't, so what?" I love this because it's so true. Some will buy from you, some won't, and either way it doesn't matter. Don't have a self-entitlement attitude; take it as experience and move on.

No one is your client until they've paid you. This is critical to remember. Sometimes hot leads will go cold; sometimes cold leads will pay you the next day. You can't predict what will happen, but I want to highlight some of the scenarios that *could* happen. You don't have a crystal ball; you don't know what could be going on in people's lives. Despite you cursing and being angry towards the hot lead that goes cold, you don't know whether they've had a death of a family member, been released by work, gotten ill, broken up with a loved one, the list continues. How would you feel if you constantly text a hot lead and they eventually replied that their mother had just passed away?

Signing people up for PT is similar to dating and finding the right partner. If you're desperate, people will pick up on this. Your mantra for personal training should always be, "They need my services more than I need their money." It's your job as an astute businessperson to make sure your finances are in order so that this is the case. Treat every single lead as neutral and follow up the hot and cold ones, but don't bank on anything. Never put all your eggs in one basket. As I said before, until there has been a transaction of funds, don't count this person as your client. Things can change in an instant. The more astute you are with your finances, the less emotional attachment you'll have to a sale.

Think of it like this. First, earn enough money to cover your outgoings for a certain amount of time. This may be gym rent, mortgage, and bills. Put this money aside for, let's say, three months. You now know that you can technically afford to turn people away if they don't meet your criteria. As long as your basics are covered, you can live without the niceties in life. Now all leads must fit your schedule and pricing, not the other way around. They must train when you can fit them in and pay what you value your sessions at. If they don't, pass them on. Self-respect is so important as a personal trainer. Unfortunately, we are seen as gym rats, juvenile trainees, and or chaperones around equipment. A lot of people *like* personal trainers, but they don't respect them. Ironically, PTs have more indirect responsibility for people's health than doctors, physicians, physios, and so on. Why? Well, who's the first person people ask for fitness and nutrition advice? What impacts the health and quality of everyone's lives? Its health and nutrition. See my point? PTs have a hell of a lot more value than they think, yet people think we'll work for peanuts and succumb to a deal if they dangle the carrot. I want you to develop a business mindset that allows you to turn these people away. You have a lot to offer, and if they don't see that then they don't deserve to work with you

Remember, no one is your client until they've paid. If people let you down, don't feel angry, sad, or like you've been hard done by. This is simply part of being in the industry. You should never succumb to pressure or people undervaluing your hard efforts. Work out your finances and spend wisely so that your basic outgoings are accounted for. Being low on finances is like swimming in a shark tank. Being desperate for money is like swimming in a shark tank with a large open wound. Your prices are your prices; your times are your times. They don't change, and if they do, you've lost your power as a businessperson and will be treated unfairly. Always set up a relationship the way you mean to go on. Give them 100%, and make sure they give you 100%. Don't give 200% and get 10% back. Dissociate yourself from the feeling that losing out on money in the short term is a bad thing. Increase the number of lead generations by delivering a great service and putting out useful content, then use this lead generation to siphon through the inquiries and find the people who perfectly fit your business. They will come. Trust me.

WHAT DICTATES YOUR HOURLY RATE

Personal training is a strange profession as there isn't a governing body that dictates how much you can charge. If someone were to have no experience in the health and fitness industry, do a six-week course, get qualified as a trainer, and charge £100 per hour, they could if they wanted to. It's a weird conundrum but one that works to your advantage. If you're unsure how much to charge or how to validate prices, this section will give you a better insight.

Conglomerate companies and gyms have a regulatory system in place for how much they pay their trainers. This usually equates to delivering a certain number of sessions, having done specific qualifications, or the duration you have been at the club. These are all valid methods of assessing rates. However, I'd like to explore what factors impact how much you charge as a self-employed personal trainer working on a freelance basis out of independent gyms. Some are more business-based, focusing on location, demographic, and P & L, while others are more internal and affected by your personal beliefs. In this chapter, I'm going to look into a few areas that play a role in hourly rate. I'm also going to discuss how you can address these factors and whether it affects your own ability to charge more.

1.   What does everybody else charge?

You may have heard the phrase, "You're the average of the five people you spend the most time with." I think that a coach charges the average of the five coaches s/he is surrounded by the most. This isn't scientifically proven, but it makes sense to me. Let's look at an example.

Say a new PT starts at your gym. The average hourly rate at your facility is £40. This PT has come in at £25. What do you think? The way I see it, you'll either assume they're not very good due to the low rates or that they're happy to undercut the more expensive coaches to get business. I'm sure if you get to know this person and became friends with them, you'd want to help them in building confidence and charging more. Over time they may increase to £30, then £35, then £40. This is because this is the standard rate at the gym. It's the norm.

Now let's look at the opposite scenario. A new trainer comes to your gym and is charging £60. This can go one of two ways. First, this rate is too expensive, the coach doesn't get clients, and has to lower their prices to get busy. Second, the coach gets clients, then other trainers get the hump and decide to increase their prices as well. What's the moral of the story? Every new addition impacts the average cost of training at that gym. They either settle into the average or the average changes. It's one or the other. This is important to consider. When working in some gyms, you can't just assess your own price, it may have to be everyone else's as well.

Of course, this will all depend on how you generate leads for your business. If you get a lot of self-generated leads, other people's pricing will not affect you. If you rely on leads from the gym, it definitely will. Price comparison is rife these days. People will always want to know the best value they can get for their money, and cheaper is better for some people.

By now you may have connected a few dots and seen where I'm going with this. You could hypothesise that as long as you are confident in creating your own leads, what you charge compared to other coaches doesn't matter, which is true. However, not everyone is at that stage yet. Generating interest from high paying clients is the holy grail of personal training. If you're able to do that, your business will grow quickly.

How is this relevant? First, if you want to charge more, you may have to consider the implications of having a higher rate. Will it make people think you have a higher skill set because you're more expensive, and therefore attract the more affluent members because they assume paying more money equals better results? Or conversely, will it deter people from working with you because of the cost and therefore reduce interest and sign up rates?

If you're looking to increase your rates, first answer these questions and brainstorm any resistance you may have in the area. If you know the average rate of what everyone is charging, would it be possible for you to annotate the average service everyone is doing too? Do they plan the sessions? Do they log the sessions? Are the actively correcting the client and coaching them or just standing there talking about their weekend? How does the client look after the session? Does the client look any different to when they started eight weeks ago? My question to you is, what do you do differently that means you're able to charge more? You can't just decide you want to be more expensive. It has to be validated or you're just making your life difficult for yourself.

I want you to be able to assess how you can increase your earnings, but I want you to work for it as well. If you do the same as everyone else, you should be charging the same as everyone else. Why's that? Think of it like this. Say you're in the market for a new car. You have a rough budget and want to get the best deal. You find the perfect car you want for £5,000 on one website and £5,500 on another. You initially don't want to break the budget but for £500 extra you get sat nav, air con, and DAB radio as standard. Because you can see the clear difference in what you pay for your money, you don't mind making that extra stretch.

If you couldn't see any difference between the cars, if it wasn't clear why one is more expensive, you'd always go for the cheaper option. Anyone would. Why would you pay more for no reason?

You can look at this from the other perspective as well. What if you found the exact car with the same specs for £4,000 on another website? The saving would be too good to miss out on, so you go for that one. If all else is equal, cheapest will win most of the time. It's only when you buy the £4,000 car and notice the small scratches on the paint work, rips in the interior fabric, and the fact it sticks when going from second to third gear that you realize why it was cheaper. Don't be offended that people look for the best deal. It's nothing against you if people opt for the cheaper option. However, most of the time, you get what you pay for. It's also important to remember that some people buy expensive cars as well. They like to treat themselves to the finer things in life and there's no reason it can't be you. In some ways, being more expensive can be an excellent sales tool as it creates hype. You gain intrigue by charging more and people want to see what the extra money buys them. The best thing about this is that if you deliver, you'll now have a referral scheme of high-paying clients.

Your number one goal as a personal trainer must be to demonstrate the value you provide. Sometimes it has to be subtle and can't be as obvious as stating your successes in your bio, but again, everything contributes. People aren't just judging you from what you write on a board or social media. People are judging you in the gym all the time. You'll be amazed how many people watch you whilst you're training people and you never realise. They are constantly evaluating what they think of you. If you charge more than the other trainers, they'll more than likely think, "Yeah okay, I can understand that." However, if they ask you what you charge but they've seen you scroll on your phone whilst a client is doing something with terrible technique, your high rates will just put them off. If we were to sit down and chat, would you be able to validate your rates based on what everyone else does in your gym? Would you be able to explain to me why you charge more? Conversely, would it be glaringly obvious that you're not charging enough for what you do? It's all relative and it all stems from the law of averages in your gym. If you want to be above the average, you need to do above average things.

2.   Geography

Your location, postcode, and local demographic play a huge role in what you charge and how you can justify it. Geography also gives you a sensible way to evaluate your business and see how you can accommodate growth. Some of the best tips I received about business actually came from the late Charles Poliquin. Despite being renowned for his strength training knowledge, I learned more about business than anything else whilst attending his seminars. When speaking about setting up a gym facility, he said that the three most important things about a gym are "location, location, location." This really resonated with me. At the time I was working in an independent facility on an industrial estate in Stockport. The gym was your typical industrial unit facility but had some great kit and great people working there. It was the first gym I worked at as a self-employed trainer. When I made the move from the commercial gym, I managed to bring some of my client base across. They were used to paying £40 an hour at the commercial gym, to which I used to get £13/15 an hour depending on how many sessions I delivered that month. As this was the case, I charged my existing clients £25 an hour to give them an incentive to move across with me. I saw it as double what I was getting at the commercial gym, so it seemed like a win.

Based on the facility I was working in, £25-35 was an accurate evaluation of what you could charge. This was because there was only one toilet, parking was available but limited, the gym got cold in the winter and boiling hot in the summer, the location wasn't easy to find, there was no spa, café, or luxurious changing facilities, and so on. Do these aspects affect what you charge per hour? It certainly did at the time. This is important to consider for any trainer unsure of whether to make the jump from commercial gym facility to independent one. Yes, you will be working for yourself, yes you will be able to charge what you want, but there will always be pros and cons to any situation. You must look at things from all angles, especially when you're young, new to the industry, and not great with business. People who train in commercial gyms are there for the luxury. If they follow you across to a gym without the luxuries they're used to, you may encounter some resistance until they see the value in the move. Please don't take this personally if they do; it's nothing against you. You just have to be conscious that moving gyms may cause an inconvenience. I'll give you an example.

Say you train Dave, a thirty-nine-year-old businessman who owns his own air conditioning company. He trains with you three times a week at your commercial gym and pays £40 an hour. He loves your sessions, finds them a great way to de-stress, and although he hasn't lost as much weight as he'd like to, he's happy with his progress so far. Dave trains with you at 5:30pm each night so he can pick the kids up from after school club on the way home from work, take them to the leisure facility, get them changed, drop them off at tennis club for an hour, then train with you whilst the kids are doing their session. Once everyone is done, they can all eat their tea in the club room. Everyone gets home tired, fed, and ready for bed by 7:30pm. Although this costs Dave a small fortune, he's happy to pay due to the convenience and the fact it makes life a lot easier. Now let's run that situation again but with Dave moving with you to an independent facility.

He may now need to ask his wife to pick the kids up from school, take them to tennis, feed them and get them home whilst he is at the gym. This isn't going to go down well. Especially as she goes to yoga at 6:00pm twice per week and will now have to miss it due to Dave's training. They compromise and Dave drops down to twice a week training with you so that he and his wife have an even share of the kid's errands. It starts with good intentions, but eventually Dave starts to get flaky, cancels a lot, and blames kids, work, and traffic.

I'm explaining this situation not so you stay at a commercial gym, but so you understand that people will pay more money for convenience. A gym's location and its ability to cater for the whole family will be more appealing to a lot of people than the quality of the trainer. I know this sounds bad but remember your demographic and target audience. They don't have the knowledge you do. You may be able to tell between a good and bad trainer, but they seldom can. Location and quality of your gym directly impacts how much you can charge. When I moved gyms in 2015, it was to a brand new, bespoke gym in a more affluent area with great parking, pristine changing rooms, and a well-stocked gym. I was able to take all my clients with me and increased everyone's rates by £5 per hour. I didn't lose any clients because they could see the difference in the facility —parking, heating, reception, shop, and cleanliness. My sessions hadn't changed, and my results hadn't changed, only the location, yet no one questioned the price increase. They could see the convenience the facility provided and so were happy to pay for it.

Here's the interesting thing. In 2016, I took the plunge and moved to a gym in Manchester City Centre, which was by far the best equipped gym I'd ever set foot in. I took two of my clients with me (as the city centre was quite far from the gym I was working in, in south Manchester) and had to rebuild my client base. Despite working in a world-class facility, I ended up dropping my prices to get busy again. Although my career took a step forward in the quality of tools I'd be using, it took a step back income wise. What's the lesson here? Clients aren't as bothered about the gym equipment they use as much as you think. When I explained to one client how much the Watson dumbbells would have cost, he replied, "Does it weigh the same as those rubber hexagon dumbbells we used to use?" I felt pretty stupid trying to justify any price increase down to kit when he put it like that.

People pay for comfort and convenience. There is absolutely nothing stopping you from charging +£50 an hour in a private facility, but you have to work pretty damn hard to build up a reputation to do so. The average person would happily pay more for an average PT in a nice gym and convenient location than an amazing one far away in an industrial unit. This is something to consider when setting up a self-employed, independent business.

3.   Postcode

This segment is about location from a socioeconomic standpoint. I'm going to include some behind the scenes "blueprint" stuff that will be extremely useful to know. The unfortunate truth with PT is that great trainers can be compartmentalised into a price bracket due to the postcode they work in. As well as the quality and convenience of the location of your gym, you must also take the surrounding area into consideration as well. This is for two reasons. First, you can always justify higher rates in more affluent areas, and second, businesspeople understand the inflation in rates due to the overheads involved.

Let's look at an example. A PT session in a gym in Mayfair London will cost you anything between £100-300 per hour. It depends on where it is and who trains you, but it's highly unlikely you'll get trained for less than three figures an hour. This may seem like a lot of money to us, but it really isn't when you consider that the average annual wage for people in this area is probably the highest in the UK and the overheads for gyms there are proportional to the amount they charge. Therefore, PTs and gym owners need to charge more to afford where they work. The exact same principle applies for the opposite end of the scale when it comes to charging lower rates. Lower income in the surrounding area equals lower rates for the PT. This will be proportional to the amount they are charged by the gym. It helps to see it in numbers, so let's have a look.

Say the average gym rent (and this is purely an estimate) in the UK is £500 in independent facilities. If the average PT session costs £35 an hour and the average delivery rate is eighty sessions a month, it works out as follows:

35 x 80 = 2800
(500/2800) x 100 = 17.8%

Therefore, with monthly fluctuations taken in to consideration, roughly 20% of a PT's income goes on gym rent. I've looked at setting up my own gym on several occasions. If you were to find a facility of around 3000 square feet in an area where the going rate for a PT is £35–40 an hour, you are looking at around £35,000 a year in rent, including business rates. This isn't taking into consideration water, gas, internet, and insurance. A decent set point to work off is around £10 per square foot for the year. This would mean the monthly rent for the facility is just under £3000, which means 4–6 trainers paying £500 a month keeps things ticking over nicely. This doesn't take into consideration paying off gym equipment, loans, utilities, and so on. So, don't think it's that simple to set up a gym. There is virtually no difference between gym facilities and house prices. As house prices go up in an area, so do the prices of any type of local facility. It's just economics. Things must be kept in balance. I could get a 5,000 square foot facility in a mill in North Manchester for the same price I'd get a 500 square foot facility in an affluent south Cheshire high street. Estate agents aren't daft, and this is a factor that affects your business.

Say some budding young fitness enthusiast wanted to set up a gym in a desirable area. It's a 3,000 square foot shop front facility with ample free parking, coffee shops, clothing stores, and gastro pubs. It's in a great location surrounded by an affluent demographic. Given everything I've already explained, how much do you think they'd be charged per square foot per year? Well, from experience and doing a lot of shopping around, I'd say they'd be extremely lucky to get it for £20, equating to £60,000 in space rent alone per year. Let's do some maths again.

£60,000 / 12 = £5000

The person is looking for six PTs to cover the rent. This means £5,000/6 = £833 per month. This is rounded up to £850 per month. Personally, I would say this is an accurate figure for the facility described. So, what does this do to the hourly rate?

We established earlier that 20% of a PT's income should go on rent. If you are paying £850 a month, your total monthly earnings would need to be £4,250 (£850 x 5). Divide this by eighty (twenty sessions per week) and the hourly rate would be £53.12, so £55 an hour rounded up for ease. Sound about right?

The gym owner then has two choices: take the rent from the PTs and rely on them getting themselves busy, or employ them as coaches, take more per hour from them, but need to provide all their trainers with business. It's an interesting conundrum that is very applicable to you. Do you do it yourself or do you let someone do it for you? It has both positives and negatives. If you are busy and pay a high amount of rent, you have the power to both increase rates and the hours you work. There's nothing stopping you from doing twenty-five sessions a week at £60 an hour and coming away with a good return. The only issue is, what happens if you're not busy or have a quiet month due to holidays or Christmas? Then you may be faced with a difficult month financially, which isn't nice. You must have the skill of knowing your finances inside out to ensure you charge what you want. If you're not as busy as you'd like and the main resistance for client uptake is pricing, you may have to re-assess your pricing structure to hit the desired delivered sessions to match your figures. You can opt for a gym that employs you; however, the biggest draw back here is being paid within their wage budget, which is usually £25-30 an hour. This is something that's never appealed to me but does come with the added security of not having to pay rent.

As you can see, there are pros and cons to everything. Business has a law of averages that works in a universal way. Most PTs charge between £30–40 an hour because their rent is around £500. To increase this, you need either to change where you work to a more desirable affluent area or build your brand, reputation, and results so you can warrant charging more in a cheaper facility. If you can't change your postcode, you need to change your brand. We'll discuss this in details in the self-development section.

4.   Education & Results

This is the area closest to my heart. As someone who loves to learn, I've always looked to re-invest money in to CPD courses. I'm not sure how much I've spent on my education. If I had to estimate, I'd say around £1500–2000 per year over the past ten years. This includes seminars, online courses, books, and other learning materials. The main reason I attended so many seminars was because I enjoyed it. I love learning and love going to educational events. It's something I'll never stop doing.

I had a big educational year in 2014. I was in my third year of uni (second time around) and invested heavily in further learning. I took a five-day seminar on programme design and kinetic chain enhancement by Charles Poliquin in Marbella, and then a four-day hypertrophy bootcamp by Andre Benoit in Southampton. If you include flights, accommodation, food, and the courses, this equated to around £7,000 in total. At the time I was charging £30 an hour on average.

This is what I wish I'd read back then: Although education is great, it needs to be looked at from a logical perspective. Does it give you the ability to enhance your product to increase demand? This is what you must ask yourself. How will said course or skill not only differentiate me from the crowd, but provide me with a skill that others don't have? The frustrating thing is that I came back from these courses motivated and educated, but in areas that bared little applicable information to my current client base. I'd spent the best part of two weeks learning about acupressure points, meridian lines, advanced hypertrophy methods, and how to train Olympic athletes. My clients were people who spent eight hours a day at a desk and couldn't figure out why they weren't losing weight despite drinking two bottles of wine a night. They weren't going to the Olympics any time soon.

If I'd presented this type of investing strategy to a business executive, they'd either laugh or cry. I'd spent 235 hours (£7000/£30) worth of working time on something that didn't contribute to the growth of my business. It was purely for interest and wanting to learn. This, from a business perspective, was pretty dumb. The problem was, at the time, I didn't think this was the case. After attending these courses, I thought I'd stretch and push my prices up to £35 for any new inquiry. I did, and I got people paying it, but it had little to do with my education and more to do with the fact I was just asking for that amount of money. There was, however, one glaringly obvious problem with my business.

I had a decent client base and averaging thirty sessions a week. I had repeat customers, people on direct debits, and knew how to train people well. The only issue was, I wasn't producing any results. I was giving out diet plans, training people well, studying daily, and generally laying the foundations of a good business. However, I never thought to broadcast transformations or 'before & afters'. This, in my opinion, is something you can't overlook. There are some great coaches out there who have never, and will never need to, post a transformation picture in their life. Their skills, knowledge, and rapport with clients will do the talking for them. This being said, some coaches are smartly use their work as ways of justifying charging above average rates, and here's the thing: people will pay it. One of my biggest objectives for this book isn't to put off aspiring PTs. It's to explain the reality of the PT world and hear the things I wish I'd heard years ago. Being integral, honest, and highly educated is a fantastic way to be. It's the only way to be in my opinion. However, if you don't know how to sell using more blunt, brash techniques, you may find resistance when increasing your fees. Think of it as being a blend between Richard Branson and Jordan Belford. Be warm, honest, and integral, but ruthless enough to sell to people to get your brand out there.

Here's me in 2014:

"Okay, so the cost of training is £35 an hour, which you can sign up for on a direct debit of £140 a month."
Potential client: "How come it's £35? Everyone else in this gym charges £25-30."
"I recently did a five-day intensive course with Charles Poliquin on neurotransmitters and the kinetic chain."'
Potential client: "Who's Charles Poliquin?"

And that, my friends, is the real world. Potential clients aren't interested in the educators we value so much. Potential clients only care about what you can do for them and whether it will be worth it. Let's compare this to alternative sales, which I know for a fact actually works. A client walks in off the back of seeing one of your transformations.

"So, what are your goals?"
Potential client: "I want to look like that latest before and after pic you put up. Would I be able to do that?"
"Yeah sure, we can use the exact same methods I did with him. If you're compliant and you work hard, you'll get those results as well."
Potential client: "How much is it?"
"£1,260 for 12 weeks training three times a week."
Potential client: "Okay, let's do it."

If you act like a business, you'll get treated like a business. People who can afford this amount for training don't care about your CPD education. Their biggest concern is getting a return for their investment. Now, there is absolutely every chance that this person may have gut, structural, or emotional issues that means a twelve-week transformation is not advisable for them, but they don't know that. After all, you didn't lie; you explained if they work hard and be compliant, they *can* get results as well. So, where does this leave us? The fact of the matter is that you are providing a product and service. Education is great but it leaves little to increasing fees if it doesn't give you anything to apply that will increase demand. Yes, it may mean you know what you're on about, but unless you're actively applying this to all your sessions day in, day out, it's not going to contribute.

My advice is to pick educational content you can use on the gym floor the next day. You must use it in a manner that means people's experience during your sessions changes. They feel like they've been worked hard, trained more efficiently, and seen a significant change. You must actively use your education to get better results. This is the best way to justify education for more money. You must do this in tandem with building better results for your business. This doesn't mean a conveyer belt of 'before and after' pictures, but a stream of people who see the benefits from your services through how you use your education.

5.   Perception of your own value

This section about your own personal belief systems and why it's holding you back in business. This is one of the most important topics in this book.

How much do you want to charge per hour? No seriously, how much would you really be happy making? Is it £5 more than what you charge now? Or £10 more? How about double? Really think about what would work well for you and your business. It requires some deep self-reflection. The way I see it, although I've been talking about what impacts hourly rate, all of it is trumped by one single factor: your own beliefs. How much you charge is comes down to how much you value yourself, and when you think about it, you are pretty damn valuable.

I know £30 an hour sounds like a lot on paper. It's almost double what the average person is paid and I'm sure many people wouldn't say no to receiving it. This being said, have you ever broken down your hourly rate and assessed why you charge that? There isn't a set formula for doing this but consider the following.

Let's say that baseline personal training is £15 an hour. This is a figure that no trainer can justify going under. It's the minimum spend, if you like. It's also the amount you're likely to get paid if you work in a commercial gym as a personal trainer. This is the rate that anyone can charge when they have qualified as a PT.

If you design sessions, turn up with a clip board or iPad, and record every weight that the person completes during their session, this comes with a service charge. I would say that this could be valued at £10 extra per session. Why? Because it's a pre-requisite for professionalism, requires extra time, and shows you have a data collection system for your clients. If someone were to buy your business from you, you could pass on your clients' training data to future trainers who could then gage where they are at. New hourly rate: £25.

Now let's say that for every year you train people, your value goes up by 5%. This is because you're spending hundreds of hours on the gym floor, building up your knowledge and experience, developing people skills, and figuring out what works and what doesn't. You make mistakes, learn from them, apply, assess, develop, apply, re-assess, develop, and so forth. If you've diligently looked to improve yourself as a coach, I would say that a 5% increase in rates is more than justifiable. If you started on £25 an hour and did this for five years, your minimum hourly rate would now be £31.90.

Let's consider education. How much CPD do you do? Every time you invest in yourself, you need to assess how you will make that money back. How much more valuable do your sessions become after attending a further learning course? What if you looked to recuperate your spends on education directly through the people who benefit from your investment, your clients?

How much did you spend on your education in the last twelve months? It's great to learn, but in business, it's all about investing to earn back with interest. As a typical interest rate is 10%, take the figure you spent on education in the past twelve months and increase it by 10%. Now take this figure and divide it by the amount of sessions you did on average last year. This will give you a figure to add on to your hourly rate for the next twelve-month phase. For example:

12-month investment in education: £2000
10% Increase: £2200
Sessions delivered last year: 960 (20 sessions per week x 48 weeks a year)
Increase for next phase: £2.29 per session

This means that with the £2.29 increase in rates, you would make your money back for the previous twelve months' worth of courses in one year. You would also make a 10% profit on this. This 10% profit is actually quite modest. If you're business minded, you may want a 15-20% return in that time. It's person dependent and the main thing is that you're looking to regain the money you invest.

So, how much are you worth now? If you've been a trainer for five years and spent at least £1,000 a year on your education, you should now be on around £37 per hour. But it doesn't end there.

How much do you do for your clients outside of the session? Although we're talking about hourly rate here, how much time per week do you put into each client with check ins, diet plans, email support, and so forth? Calculate this in hours per week, multiply by your hourly rate, and divide by the amount of sessions per week you do. For example:

3 hours client admin per week
Hourly rate: £37
Extra work: 3 x 37 = £111
Sessions per week: 20
Cost of extra work: £5.55 recuperated per session
New hourly rate: £42.55

Still think you're only worth £30 an hour?

The truth is, it doesn't work *exactly* like this. You can charge whatever you like in theory, it just depends on your confidence and self-belief. A lot of personal trainers undervalue themselves and worry about what people will think of them if they increase their rates. In reality, all you are doing is short-changing yourself. When you assess the work you put in, you actually do a lot, and you do need to be paid for it. My goal here isn't to provide arbitrary data so that you can present all this info to clients and tell them your rates are going up. People will pay what you ask for if you present yourself with enough assertiveness. I just want you to finish this section, put the book down, take a deep breath, and say aloud: "I am good at what I do and I work hard to help people. I deserve to be paid well for it." It's not that personal training needs to be affordable; it's that you need to communicate with people so that they find your services incredibly valuable.

Think of things like this. The Pikachu Illustrator Pokémon card was first published in 1997 with only six copies printed. As it is so rare and sought after, one Pokémon fanatic paid an incredible $100,000 for the card on eBay. Just let that sink in: over triple the average annual salary on a small baseball card with a picture of a yellow mouse on it. Would you pay that? It may depend on both how much you earn and how much you like Pokémon, but my guess is that if you won the lottery tomorrow, it wouldn't be the first thing on your list. Do you think the person who bought this card got a good deal or a bad deal?

The way I see it, there are three possible outcomes in business: good, bad, and neutral. The result is largely dependent on negotiation skills and the perception of value from those who are doing the transaction. Say you are the one selling the Pokémon card. You know that it's worth at least $75,000, so you ask for $100,000 with the intent of getting knocked down. There are now three ways this can go. The buyer may agree to $100,000 immediately. They may value the card so highly and have been looking for it for so long that they're happy to pay whatever it takes to secure the purchase. This is a good transaction for the seller. In another scenario, the buyer may not agree on the price, negotiate with the vender, and they agree on $75,000. This is a neutral transaction as both parties have made an exchange for what they perceive to be an accurate evaluation of the item. Finally, we have the situation where the purchaser puts an initial offer of $50,000 on the table. The vender now must explain why they couldn't justify selling the card for that amount. If they do succumb to the pressure and agree to the offer, this would be a bad outcome for them. The take home point here is that as mentioned before, negotiation skills and perception of value are without a doubt the biggest factors that dictate how much you charge per hour. You must have a set figure you're not willing to go under and you must be able to demonstrate value so the person understands why it's set at this amount.

As the years go by and we gain experience, knowledge, and a reputation, it's important we look to increase our perceived value in ourselves. In other words, the minimum amount you'd take for the Pokémon card. It's a step by step process and not something you can do overnight. It takes time and effort. When I went from working in a commercial gym to self-employed, what I earned per hour jumped from £13 to £25. This was massive for me and incredibly exciting at the time. I remember the first month I broke the £2,000 mark in earnings. I felt like I'd won the lottery. The problem was, clients had been paying me £40 an hour at the commercial gym, and therefore I knew my time was worth more than what I was charging. It took me two years to go from £25 to £40 an hour on a self-employed basis, and this is what I want people to understand. Just like anything, you have to be patient and consistent. Jumping the gun in business is risky. It may work but it may not. Price increases are only warranted once you've earned the right through quality of service and reaching capacity. This must be done in tandem with a shift in mindset and constantly reiterating to yourself what you're worth.

HOW TO STRUCTURE A
CONSULTATION

We've established that people need a personal trainer and
that there's a market for it. We're now going to delve in to how
to present training packages. We'll be covering how you
communicate your services to a client and make them want to
work with you, how you get them to sign up for high frequency
training, and how to structure your training plans so that all
outcomes suit your business but keep the clients best interest
in mind.

Don't sell, solve.

I don't believe in selling; I believe in problem solving and
presenting your product. You could argue that this is essentially
the same thing, but it depends on your agenda. I think selling
indicates that you're more concerned about the exchange of
money. It can be construed as a dirty word and that the main
objective is for a transaction to occur. If this is the case, I don't
want you to sell at all. I want you to display your services and
be selective over who you work with. You must reiterate to
yourself that you are helping people, your services are
improving people's lives, and that the money they pay you in

return is a justified fee for the value you've brought them. The more you believe this, the more natural selling your services should feel.

Cast your mind back to what I said in the beginning of the book. I've seen many great salespeople personal trainers who have no problems at all getting busy. They just have huge issues retaining clients, training them well, and building a good reputation. Being good at selling is just a small part of business development. If there is no foundation to your services, systems, and desire to help people, you simply won't grow. Be wary of any product that offers to help you with your sales skills alone. Sales is just confidence in your product and conviction during delivery. It's not about using fancy language, special techniques, or subliminal messaging. You can't trick people into working with you. I genuinely believe that everyone would benefit from a personal trainer. Your goal is to show people where they've been going wrong, why it's impacted their results, and what you bring to the table to solve this problem. Your goal during a consultation should be to get the person talking. You want them to tell you things that you can pick up and then ask them to explain in more detail. The skill of listening is critical during initial interactions. If you just talk about what you have to offer, it may not fit in with what the person needs. If you listen to their needs and explain how you solve their problems, your value goes up. Let's take a look at a couple of scenarios.

Scenario 1 - You do the talking

Trainer: "I have done four courses this year in nutritional programming, biomechanics, and NLP. I got a first in sports science at university and currently compete to a national level in powerlifting. I'm confident in my methods and I am sure you'll be able to lose two stone in weight whilst working with me."

I'm sure none of you would sell like this, but my point is that highlighting credentials does little to entice a client into working with you. Here you are actively trying to sell by telling them about your value, but it's too cryptic. You may have these impressive accolades, but it doesn't mean anything to the client. What can you do for them?

<u>Scenario 2 - They do the talking and you problem solve</u>

Trainer: "What have you done in the past and did it work well for you?"

Potential Client: "I tried the Atkins diet and that initially worked very well, but I started to get cravings really badly in the afternoon and eventually gave in. I ended up putting on more weight than I lost after I finished the diet. I don't know why, but I can't seem to stop eating carbs. My main goal is to lose a bit of weight, so I run 2–3 times per week. I had to stop this though as I got really bad shin splints. I haven't done much exercise since."

At this point, you should be taking notes and looking at which bit of information you wish to explore further.

Trainer: "Where did you get the idea about the Atkins diet?"

Potential Client: "Everyone at work was going on about it and how well it worked. Lindsey in accounts said she lost two stone in eight weeks on it. I just couldn't do it; I found myself going dizzy and snacking once I got home."

How much information have you taken away from this small interchange? I can tell you now, a hell of a lot. The courses you've done, the degrees you've obtained, and competitions you've placed in mean nothing in this situation. You need to show this lady how your services can be the solution to all her problems. You need to be positive, helpful, and highlight her mistakes carefully without making her feel like she's wasted time. Your goal here isn't to show off how much you know, it's to explain how much you'll be able to help her. A big mistake I used to make during consultations was trying to over complicate things. I thought that the person thinking I was smart would make them want to work with me. If anything, I'd lose them and make it look like I wasn't listening. It is key to listen to them intently and address their specific issues. Highlight where you think they're going wrong and then look to discuss it further.

"The Atkins diet is a sound method, but all it has done is take carbs out of your diet. Carbs aren't bad for you in the right amounts, you were probably just consuming too many calories through carbs. If you eat something in high amounts, taking them out completely will leave your body wondering where they've gone. That's why cravings are completely normal. My goal would be to keep carbs in your diet, but in the right amount and within a calorie-controlled diet based on your weight, activity levels, and goals. Have you ever used MyFitnessPal?"

Don't worry if during a consultation you say things that aren't technically perfect. It's important that *you* understand biochemical mechanisms, hormones, and micronutrients, but when speaking to potential clients, you must speak to them in a way they understand. You want them to realise that you've worked with a plethora of people just like them and helped them get results too. Your experience will impress them, not necessarily your knowledge. The goal of a consultation is to show how you are the solution to the specific problems they have. Let's take the woman in this example. From this short interchange you'll have deciphered that she struggles with her weight, is heavily influenced by what other people at work say, has a poor relationship with food, and doesn't have the best of routines. This is where you come in.

"Our goal will be to establish a routine where you never allow the hunger pangs to set in. If you usually feel ravenous at 4:00pm, we'll look to have a small snack at one or two, whether it's a small piece of fruit or cereal bar. Snacks are fine as long as you track them all and they fit within your calorie allowance. We'll need to balance out your calories so you're eating a higher amount of protein. By looking at your food diary, you're getting around 60–70g a day at the moment. We'd like that to be around 120g, but that might not be realistic initially, so let's aim for 100g first. I can

break this down for you so it's spread across four manageable meals throughout the day."

Highlight where they are going wrong, devise a plan of action, and explain how you can help. You can do this for any problem they're having. Typical sales are outcome based: "If you train with me, you'll lose two stone, become fitter, and love your body." You're selling them the dream not the answer. I want you to provide solutions for people during your consultations that make them see that not using your services would be a mistake. How do you become a necessity? It's not by selling, it's by solving. Beginning any consultation by asking them for the top three things they've struggled with whilst losing weight would be an excellent starting point. You can simply spend the rest of the time listening to the person and discussing how you can help them.

I seldom speak in absolutes, but I will say this: once a week personal training doesn't work. Let's look at it from this perspective: Is high frequency personal training more effective? Yes, it certainly is. Therefore, it makes sense from a business perspective to push your more efficient training strategy. All your clients are paying for results in some format. If training more gets them better results, you should encourage them to train as much as possible. Would they have a better training session if you were there? Absolutely. You would be on hand to motivate them, count reps, time rest intervals, spot them, correct technique, and tell them what weight to use. A training session is improved tenfold by having an attentive trainer on hand. Your goal during a training session is to train someone so well, they realise they wouldn't be able to achieve the same training effects without you. Remember, necessity, not nicety. The more "untrained" someone is, the more they need a trainer with them. If they have poor mobility, poor body awareness, and are low on confidence, they will likely either skip the gym or play it safe and opt for the cardio equipment. I would say that the lower the training age, the more frequent PT they need. I know what you're thinking: "Yeah, I agree, but what about money? A lot of my clients can't afford training with me that much." I totally get it, so let's look at solutions.

Firstly, once a week PT is not once a week. If you want people to get results, you'll have to write a training plan for 2–3 other sessions in the gym that week as well. This takes time and effort. As you don't see them that regularly, you'll also have to check in with them via text or email to keep them on track. Without that daily reminder of having you there to talk about nutrition and habit formation, it can be easy for them to slip back into old ways. Suddenly that one hour a week they've purchased starts to stretch a bit further. With programme design and contact time, you have to set aside at least another hour to help them. This effectively halves your hourly rate. If they're paying £40 for once per week, it starts to look more like £20 per unit of time. Time is always money. Low frequency PT is not only an inferior way of getting results, it's also an inefficient way of earning money. Here are two options I recommend.

Option 1 - Remove the once per week option

I've gotten some great results with people, which I'm proud of. These people trained 3–5 times a week with me to achieve these results. Frequency is key and if people are serious about making a change, they need to see you regularly. If you're an established PT and are doing at least fifteen sessions a week consistently, I would remove your once a week training options. You know people won't get results doing once per week, so why sell an inferior product? If you know something isn't going to work, utilising it is bad for business. The last thing you want is for someone to buy a block of ten sessions off you, not see any change, and leave ten weeks later looking no different. This has happened to me and so I needed to find ways to change it. I recommend presenting your packages in blocks of eight or twelve. You state that you have a minimum of twice a week commitment, as this is the best way to get results. You are the businessperson and you create the terms. If they buy eight sessions, they will be with you for at least a month. If they buy twelve and like what you have to offer, it's likely they'll increase to three times a week and continue with you in that fashion from there. To make this even more tangible for the client, you could reduce your block of twelve prices by 10–20% to entice them that way.

Option 2 - Make once a week much more expensive

As already discussed, once per week personal training is a lot of work. If you're spending more time outside of the session to ensure the person has the support they need, you're diluting your income. If you increase your fees for once a week PT by 1.25–1.5 your normal hourly rate, it's a win–win situation. Say you value your time at £35 an hour. You could even calculate your time precisely if you have the appropriate data. Find out your average hourly rate by adding up what all your clients pay per hour and dividing by how many clients you have. If you're busy and financially stable, multiply this figure by 1.5 and then use this as a marker for your new once a week rate. This means if you're charging £30 per session on average, once a week PT is now £45. The question now is, how do you present this?

A block of ten sessions is as arbitrary as ten reps. Just as reps are relative to the goal, so is how many sessions you sell. If you've had great success using the ten-block method, then well done. I'm not saying it is wrong, but it doesn't stipulate a designated period. Four, eight, and twelve sessions could be once or twice a week from anywhere from 4–6 weeks. Ten is neither here nor there. It's twice a week for five weeks or three times a week for three and a third weeks. In my mind, that just doesn't make sense. As well as this, what if the person opts to do three times a week with you? They're now paying the same as someone training once per week. There's no "discount" for increased frequency, therefore in their eyes no incentive to train more often. I use the word discount but what I really mean is encouragement. Your goal should be to get the person to train as much as possible with you. Why? For better results and greater spend.

Say you sold your packages in monthly blocks. These are packs of four, eight and twelve. People buy via BACS transfer initially and can then move on to direct debit after one month. I'm asking you now, if you wanted value for money, which one would you buy?

Block of 4: £180
Block of 8: £300
Block of 12: £360

Do the maths and training three times per week gets you 33% off the initial hourly rate. That's quite the discount. In this person's eyes, they're getting a £45 trainer for 2/3 of the price. "Hang on, Chris, you've spoken in great detail about perception of value and not short changing yourself. Aren't you under cutting yourself by only charging £30 an hour?"

Yes, you would be. However, if you make your three times a week option the equivalent of your current average hourly rate, you're no worse off. Therefore, a golden rule here is that once you are filling up and stable, change your package structures to promote people training with you more frequently. You are only worth the price of your cheapest client. If new clients are paying £40 an hour, but you still have a client who has been with you for three years paying £30, your average rate will be in the low £30s. Your data won't lie; that's why tracking everything is so important. Your goal here is to make high frequency training the most logical option. If it gets better results and it's more cost effective, why wouldn't they go for it? People also (generally) like to train at the same time. How would five people training at the same time Monday, Wednesday, and Friday, and five people training at the same time Tuesday and Thursday sound to you? You have routine and a set diary and bring in £3,300 a month on a direct debit. Stability potentiates the ability for growth. Once you've maintained this level of income for 3–6 months, you can then focus on the next phase, which would be to increase prices. Some may stay, some may leave, but you have systems in place, and more importantly free time, to dedicate to increasing brand awareness.

PAYMENT METHODS

Payment methods weren't covered in my PT course. I'd love to know if it's something they now talk about openly and educate trainers on the best methods in which to arrange transactions. This chapter will explore the pros and cons of both options and which one may be better suited to you.

Direct Debits

I'm a big fan of direct debits. I see the accumulation of DD clients as building up my own wage and security. Direct debits are great as they take away the hassle for the client. Once sent up, you don't have to have any awkward conversations about money or asking for payments, which makes your life a lot easier. Most clients will see the PT direct debit as an area of their income that is accounted for. For example, if they earn £4,000 a month, £320 goes out on training twice a week with their trainer. It's under 10% of their income so nothing too drastic.

Direct debits are good to push towards well organised, prompt people who are number and data orientated. This is not based on science or psychology, it's purely my own observation. You could also argue that DDs are good for people who are the exact opposite. They're poorly organised so it's better if they don't have to think about regular payments. However, you may struggle to get these people to set up the standing order or DD in the first place. The people I've had on DDs are usually the ones who are good with figures (accountants, lawyers, and analysts) and also like seeing the data from their sessions and biofeedback—lifting loads, calories, macros, heart rate, HRV, etc. If you have people who have been with you for longer than six months and you know they're happy with your services, I strongly recommend getting them set up on a direct debit or standing order for the first of each month. It can be whichever date you choose, but doing it after payday is wise. This tends to be the 28th of each month for most people. Direct debits take away getting frustrated when a client says they're going to pay but don't. A lot of the time people aren't malicious, they just forget. Personally, I hate sending those prompting to pay messages to clients, which is why direct debits are great. It makes things easier for everyone.

I wouldn't say there are that many cons to direct debits, especially if you've had the client a while. However, some issues can arise with new clients when it comes to seeing whether they've actually set up a direct debit or they've just made a one-off payment. I've had it a couple of times where people have made the bank transfer for the first instalment, but sent it as a single transfer and not set up a DD. If this happens, prepare yourself for a flaky client. These people also tend to be the ones who pay late. Here's an example of what I've experienced in the past.

Me: Please set up your DD to come out on the first of each month. The amount is £200 for four sessions a month.

Person: Okay, no problem, will do.

You do your first session on the 3rd of that month and you still haven't received a payment. As the client seems like a nice trusting person, you text them during the week again asking for them to set up the DD.

"Yep, will do."

They come in for the next session on the 10th (still not having made the payment) and say, "Can I pay by cash, please?" You being a nice person say, "Yeah, that's fine this month, but could you please set the payment up for the beginning of next month?"

It may not be any shock to you that these people only do 1–2 months with you, max. They drop off, don't lose any weight, and don't get anywhere. It's like their apprehension to making a commitment is their own block and they're scared to actually set up a proper payment plan because it means they'll indefinitely have to go to the gym. This is, in my opinion, the downfall of direct debits: no buy in. If people are fearful of commitment, direct debits will scare them. These are usually the people who are doing PT for the first time in their lives. To simplify things, look to convert anyone who's been training with your consistently for over three months on to a direct debit. This will make things much easier for you and them. For new clients, the goal is just to get them training so that they can see the benefit in your service.

Up Front Payments

Getting an upfront payment for training sessions is great. Not only does it mean you'll be working for someone for a while, it also gives you some financial security for a few months. If your gym rent is £500 a month, and you sell a block of thirty-six sessions for £1,260, training just one client three times a week has sorted your overheads at the gym for two and a half months. The package people will prefer may depend on the personality type. Business owners or corporate types who are a little desensitised to money wouldn't think twice about dropping a couple of grand in one go. After all, that's not a great deal of money to them. We as trainers assume that £50 an hour is a lot of money and asking for it in a block of thirty six is obscene. However, there are some business owners that will spend quadruple that on their office Christmas party and not think twice about it. Money is relative. That's the most important thing you need to know about selling. If you're fishing in the right pond, big fish will bite.

One thing I must stress when it comes to up-front payments is responsibility. If you get several hundred or thousands of pounds in advance, don't treat it any differently to how you would with your other payment plans. No holidays, no fancy clothes, no lavish treats. Just put it straight in the bank and be sensible. Trust me on this one. Although it's more business-like to secure a big up-front payment, there are several cons, the first being the obvious one of asking for a lot of money. If Jane from Weight Watchers has been seeing a PT once a week for the past two years and paying £120 a month in cash, she'd be mortified when you quote her for £1,260 in the consultation. It will straight up scare the living daylights out of people. Another downside to upfront payments is that you may have to go cheaper. If your hourly rate is £35, people may automatically assume that the more they buy from you, the cheaper you'll be. Some people might even see this as an opportunity.

You: It's £35 for one-off sessions, or you can buy a block of thirty sessions for £900

Them: Okay, would it be possible for you to do fifty sessions for £1,000?

A grand there and then? Sounds hard to pass on, doesn't it? Especially when you're used to getting £300-400 here and there. Go on then, sounds good. What's the problem? You're now working for £20 an hour. Never, ever do this. Don't ever go lower than 25% of what you would charge for one hour of your time, no matter how many sessions you sell. If your hourly rate is £35 an hour, you never go below £26, even if you sold a hundred sessions in one go. Stick to that rule.

A big part of judging whether you should present your packages as a direct debit or up-front payment is knowing your demographic. If you work close to the city centre and have more affluent clientele, a large payment may be easier for the client as they only have to think about payments once every three months. It reduces their to-do list and means an area of their life is boxed off for the next twelve weeks. If you're in a rural area and your clientele aren't business executive types, the direct debit option is probably more advisable. The best option is whatever you feel comfortable with. Print all your packages out in to a clearly presented PDF or leaflet for the person to take away with them. This way they can go home and assess their best options. Don't be afraid to trial and error packages and see what works best for you. You may find that all your clients go for up-front packages and so this becomes the norm to you. Alternatively, you may get an adverse reaction to asking for thousands of pounds and so be deterred from trying that option again. This isn't a mistake in business, it's a learning curve. The most important thing is that you're able to negotiate an hourly fee that reflects your quality of service. Let's look at an example.

"Sessions are bought in blocks of thirty-six for an up-front payment of £1,260."

The client gulps and looks worried. They're keen to work with you but weren't expecting to spend that much money.

"If the up-front payment is too much of a commitment, you could opt for the monthly instalments of £480."

This is virtually a third of your initial proposal. Suddenly it seems like the more logical option for the person. The great thing about this is that it actually works out at more per hour for you. Never get short sighted by the opportunity to get more money in one go; always look for the option that means you earn more per hour. This is ultimately your wage. In an ideal world you would charge what you want per hour in an up-front payment with no exceptions. Present them with a descending payment scheme that gets less intimidating as you go.

12 Week Block - 36 sessions £1260
4 Week Block - 12 sessions £480
Monthly Online Training - £100 per month

If you've impressed this person with your level of knowledge, they'll want to work with you. You just need to present them with packages that mean you win regardless of what they choose to go for. The most important thing is that they have options (but not too many) so that you don't lose them. Up-front payments mean a win for you as you get a lot of money in advance, job security, and know you'll be working with the client for a sufficient period. Direct debit adds to you monthly DDs and you get more money per hour. With online training, the client stays with you in some format but this time with a product that doesn't take up too much of your time. This would be an awesome one to have as an option if you work in a commercial gym. Your sign-up process should suit you, not necessarily the client. Remember, during consultations, what's the worst thing that could happen? They don't sign up. That's nothing at all against you; just move on to the next lead and do not be deterred. If you are a good trainer, they missed out, not you. The most important thing is that you are relaxed and authoritative during an interaction. They may not sign up now, but if they like you and can see you know your stuff, it doesn't mean they won't sign up in the future. Anybody in a gym could be your client, even if they (or you) don't know it yet.

Although it may seem like generating leads and signing people up is what creates income, it is actually represented by session delivery rate. Once someone buys a block off you, they can't buy another block until their current one is finished. Therefore, it's in your best of interests to get them to complete the sessions in the shortest time possible. If you're a one-to-one trainer, you only earn money when you're working. This section will talk you through why terms and conditions and having a thorough, well explained cancellation policy is a business essential.

Every time a client's sessions take longer than expected to end, you are losing money. If you have thirty slots per week designated for training people and a three time a week a client cancels all their sessions for a fortnight, you lose out on income unless you can quickly fill the same slot. It's possible for this to happen but seldom easy. Even if you have a waiting list, you need the person to be able to fit in with the times available. This is why you have to lay foundations that protect your business. If you work in a commercial gym, it's likely that the club requires you to get your client to fill in a T & C's form as a mandatory procedure prior to training. I recommend you carry over the same practises you have in a commercial setting to your self-employed business. Regardless of where you work, get the client to sign a contract you have written. If you don't feel confident in what to write, there are a tonne of resources online that can show you standard terms for personal training contracts. There's nothing wrong in using these templates and adjusting them to your own preferences. You can state your designated working times, what you expect from the client, and your stance on cancellations. Not only are you creating a much safer foundation to you to work in, doing this screams professionalism and shows you are serious about business. I recommend getting the client to read through the T & C's, signing them once they are happy, and then photocopying the contract and giving them both a physical and scanned online version to keep themselves. It's critical that you lay foundations as early as possible. Be it calorie baselines, movement quality, or cancelation periods, the client need to know what's expected of them.

The standard cancellation policy is usually twenty-four hours' notice. This means that if someone were to notify you that they can't make the session within twenty-four hours of the session itself, they will be charged the full amount. If you don't have set T & C's given to you by a commercial gym, this is what I recommend you put in your own contracts. This being said, there is obviously a level of common sense needed when it comes to the cancellation policy. If you are too stern, you'll risk losing the client. If you are too lenient, you risk people taking advantage of you. You have to find a sweet spot between both understanding and authoritative. It's tricky and does come with experience. I can tell you now if you have a new client who's just started with you and they text you are 8:30am saying they can't make it to their session at 8am the next day, quoting your twenty-four hour cancellation policy wouldn't be wise. How the person reacts will largely depend on their personality type; however, it's always important to think, "How would I feel if put in the same situation?" Your goal is to build rapport with your client so that they trust you. Clients who trust you will train with you for longer. Being too stern may make you seem a little too money conscious. A little common sense does go a long way. In general, the closer to a session a client cancels, the more valid your choice is to charge them.

You always have to consider how you protect both your time and income. A thorough cancellation policy does both. However, I wouldn't just include it in a contract; I would speak to the client before you've even stepped foot on the gym floor. Growth is all about getting uncomfortable. Just as it's important to deliver your session prices in a calm and relaxed manner whilst retaining eye contact, you should do the same when stating your policies to cancellations. Make sure the client is completely okay with this and have a conversation about it.

If you get a client to sign a contract without talking the conditions through, there's every chance they could turn around to you and say, "I wasn't aware of that." Unfortunately, some people can get funny and protective when it comes to losing out on money. You may have a client who seems like a lovely person, yet you really see the ugly side of them when you charge them for a last-minute bail. Never give them the opportunity to say that something wasn't made clear. I've made this mistake in the past and want to ensure that no trainer who reads this ever does it themselves. It's awkward and can be testing during the early stages of your career. Get people to read the contract, get them to sign it, then clearly speak to them about the contract. You must say, "As you'll have read, all sessions cancelled within a twenty-four-hour period are charged the full amount. Are you okay with this?" Most people will say yes, but if someone does say no, as they may be subject to last minute changes in their schedule on a regular basis. Make sure you discuss this issue with them and come up with a solution.

You may be thinking, "Okay, got you, but what if they have to cancel for a really legitimate reason? Where does that leave us?" Again, this all boils down to common sense. If you get a text saying, "Can't make it to tonight's session. My grandma has just passed away and the whole family is devastated," don't tell them they will be charged for the session. This is a sure-fire way of losing business and being brandished an insensitive money grabbing (insert profanity of your choice here). However, if it's 6:30pm and you get a text from your 7:00pm client saying, "Sorry, work is manic. Won't be able to make it tonight," you must explain the situation there and then. "Thanks for letting me know. Just so you're aware, I will need to charge due to late cancellation." This text goes one of two ways. The person is either completely fine with it and books in for their next session, or they challenge your statement. If you can say, "As you'll remember during our consult, all sessions come with a twenty-four-hour cancellation policy. This will be clearly stated on the hard copy of my T & C's and the email version I sent to you." If you don't say that, you technically don't have a leg to stand on. If your client happens to be an executive or lawyer, they'll take you to the cleaners. Don't risk fighting battles you can't win because of a lack of organisation.

Cancellations are a funny area. Any seasoned PT will tell you this. I've had people who've bought a block of ten sessions, turned up for two of them, then immediately bought another block of ten and continued in the same fashion. I've also had people who get their diaries out and send you a complete record of the completed sessions as soon as you reference a late cancellation. As the old saying goes, there's nowt queer as folk (apologies to any non-British readers who have no idea what that means) but in a nut shell, it all depends on who you're working with. The most important thing is that you have some terms and conditions for them to sign, you give them both a signed hard copy and email scan, you speak about your cancellation policy in person with them prior to starting sessions, and that you are thorough and consistent when charging for no shows.

A little bonus tip would be to write in your intentions to implement a price increase in to your terms and conditions. I can appreciate that you may think it'll put potential clients off, but if it's worded correctly it'll show that you're astute with your business model. People will respect that. You can also state that your price increases are justified by your reinvestment in your business. So for example;

My Personal Training rates are subject to a 5% increase on 1st March each year. This is given that I have met your expectations of professionalism and results and attended at least 2 CPD courses in a 12 month time frame.

Keeping it short and sweat is sufficient. Your clients will get to know you and respect your desire to better yourself. Having it written down in the initial terms and conditions sets foundations and is very important, especially if the client stays with you long term. Remember; it's your average hourly rate, not necessarily your highest hourly rate that you need to work on.

RESULTS EFFICIENCY

Are you frustrated by your lack of results with clients? Do you often question your methods and whether you're any good as a trainer because you don't have a huge catalogue of before and afters? What if I was to tell you it has less to do with what you're doing with the person and more to do with how often you're training the person? Let's discuss.

According to the Guinness Book of World Records, the largest pumpkin ever grown weighed over 1,190 kg. That's roughly three fifths as heavy as your average car. Pretty impressive, right? How do I know this and why is it relevant? Well, you have a man named Mike Michalowicz to thank for that. In his excellent 2012 book, *The Pumpkin Plan*, Mike explains how business owners were able to grow their profits through using the same methods prize-winning pumpkin farmers used to grow these insanely sized jack-o-lanterns. First he explains the principles behind the strategy and then talks about different case studies that have yielded great results. Whilst I was listening to the book on Audible, I was waiting with bated breath to hear him talk about an example in the personal training industry. Unfortunately, he didn't, which is why I'm going to cover it for you now.

The Pumpkin Plan is basically about spotting earlier potential and doing everything you can to make sure this potential develops. You do this by weeding any smaller, undeveloped pumpkins away from the vicinity of the thriving pumpkin and ensuring nothing can interfere with its growth. It doesn't stop there though; nurturing is only half of the equation, and nature plays a big role too. These pumpkins need not only the right environment, but also the right genetics. To grow a massive pumpkin, you need a seed that comes from a massive pumpkin. Farmers have been known to pay incredible amounts for just one seed from these orange abnormalities. It's the genetic coding in the seed that gives you the best chance of growing your own monstrous overgrown squash yourself.

What can you take from this? Well, if you want a business that gets amazing results and is a perpetual internal referral scheme, you need to Pumpkin Plan your business. You do this by laying the correct foundations and removing distractions or other components that get in the way of development. As a trainer, there's nothing more exciting than when someone "gets it" and suddenly understand macros and calories and become extremely compliant. Every time they come in, they've lost weight and you can see the physical difference in them each week. They're ecstatic with their results and constantly thank you for your help. It's an amazing feeling. Conversely, I'm sure we all know the feeling of the client who constantly makes excuses. They cancel, they're late, they never fill in their food diary and spend most of their sessions complaining about work, their spouse, or the weather. Ultimately, they just leave you feeling frustrated and as if you're a bad trainer. Now what happens if this client happens to be booked in just before your thriving client? You have a client who's doing incredibly well, getting results, and singing your praises, but your session delivery is subpar because you've just had the life sucked out of you by an energy vampire. This is an example of something that needs weeding to put focus into a greater project. You need to Pumpkin Plan your business. So, how do you do this?

In situations like this, the most important thing to remember is respect and choice of wording. How you communicate to people is essential and incorrect language could be detrimental to your business and reputation. This being said, you need to explain to your non-compliant, frustrating client that if they don't improve their diligence, they are just wasting their money with you. If you're polite and honest, people will respect you. Saying, "Look, I appreciate work is stressful at the moment, but you haven't lost any weight in eight weeks. I feel like I'm just taking your money right now, which isn't right. I'm happy to put sessions on hold for now or look at online options so you're not wasting your money." I've had chats like this with clients on many occasions. It's a sensitive conversation, but one that needs to be had. No, it's definitely not firing your clients—this is a rude and nonsensical notion. It's merely explaining to them that they are not getting the maximum return for their investment and this is what business is ultimately about. One thing you have to make peace with as a personal trainer is that despite your knowledge and expertise, some people won't get the best results purely because of their lifestyle. It's not your fault and it's not necessarily theirs.

A huge part of being a good trainer is managing lifestyle, not trying to completely overhaul it. Once this client realises that you're just looking out for their best of interests (and their bank account) they may opt to leave the sessions or go to your online services. You don't want to lose them as a client, you just want to ensure they're not interfering with your ability to get awesome results with your prize pumpkin. It sounds ruthless, but there's absolutely nothing more powerful in the personal training industry than word of mouth referrals. You can have all the social media followers you want, but it's superfluous to when someone says to their friend, "You need to go and see them. They're amazing, I lost three stone with them and loved the training." People can't say this if you're not performing to your best. You must put energy into what's thriving.

That's the nurture side of things covered, now what about the nature? Although it's not possible to send all potential clients to 23 and Me to check if they have great genetics for muscle building and fat loss, it is possible to create a better environment for success from the get-go. Having a good "seed" is someone who understands what you want them to do and why you want them to do it from the start. Honesty is essential. If people want to lose a lot of body fat in a short period of time, they need to understand that cardio and dietary adherence will be paramount. You can't pull the wool over their eyes. The reality is, rapid results do take an incredible level of sacrifice and dedication. If someone comes to you and says that's what they want, it's your job to make them fully understand what they're in for. To create your perfect seed, you need to get into their head, find out their why, explore their obstacles, and provide solutions.

This is also a situation where you can't be afraid to up-sell. If you get a highly motivated client, it's your job to increase frequency and give them the best chance of achieving exceptional results. Results equal referrals and referrals mean growth.

I split my years up into phases. Each phase is a three-month period also known as a quarter. When I first ventured in to delivering seminars, I needed to be efficient with my time in order to write the content out for the courses. As this was the case, between January and March 2018 I only had five clients. It doesn't sound like much, but it becomes relative when you consider each client saw me four times a week in the same time slot. I worked Monday, Tuesday, Thursday, and Friday, taking Wednesday and weekends off for content development. My clients saw me at 7:00, 9:00, and 10:00am and then 4:30 and 5:30 in the evening. I'd use the quiet time in the day to train, eat, and write the slides and handbooks for the seminars. It was tough and felt like Groundhog Day a lot of the time, but it worked. If I sat down with a trainer and they told me they had 15–20 clients, I'd be impressed with their ability to sign people up, but not with their business model. Having a high volume of clients is inefficient and I can show you why with maths.

Effort and income are only proportional to each other if every single client brings in the same amount of money. If you have ten clients and they all pay you £40 a session and all train with you twice per week, then 10% of your effort brings you 10% of your income. The thing is, this is rare in business. Upon review, you'll probably notice some anomalies and areas where it would make sense to maximise. For example, say you have that once per week client who's not getting anywhere. They've been with you for four years, still haven't lost any weight, and train once per week paying £30 an hour. Compare this to a new star client you have. They train with you three times per week at £40 an hour and are raving to the high heavens about your services. If your average income is £3,000 per month, the statistical break down of what each client returns looks like this. Your once a week client works out at 4% of your return (120/3000) whereas your three times a week clients works out at 16% of your return (480/3000).

Here you have a disproportionate distribution of effort to return. As personal trainers, a client represents a percentage of our time and headspace dedicated to helping people achieve results. If we keep things simple and say the trainer in this example has ten clients, you have one 10% that is worth four times more than another. If we applied the Pumpkin Plan to this situation, we would weed away the low-returning 10% and feed the high-returning 10%. You could do this by:

- Explaining to your once per week client paying £30 per hour that personal training isn't for them given their level of commitment right now;
- Increase their hourly fees from £30 to £40 so it brings up your average hourly rate;
- Explain that they'll see better results if they increase one to one training frequency to 2–3 times per week; or
- Move them towards your online services.

In tandem with this, you could say to your client training three times a week that their results would be even better if they moved up to four times per week. If they did, you'd drop their hourly rate slightly (as an incentive) to £37.50 an hour, meaning they now pay £600 per month. From a business perspective, you've just shifted the ratio of client to return in your favour. You've reduced your client workload but increased one client from a 16% return to a 20% return. Same money, less work, smarter model. Astute business is about clearing out deadwood and feeding areas with the greatest potential for growth. I fully appreciate that people aren't just stats and you have relationships and report built with them. However, there needs to come a point where you take a step back, assess the situation, and really evaluate what's going on. It's common for people to use a personal trainer as a means of *feeling* like they're committed to fitness. By paying someone to train them, it's a way of convincing themselves that they are taking the necessary steps to be healthy. In reality, they haven't prioritised their lifestyle, habits, or focus to change their physique at all. They've created a scapegoat that provides the illusion of wanting to change.

We've now entered a unique situation that I believe is bespoke to personal training. It's where people pay you but receive no return for their investment. If you go to a barber and he does a great job of cutting your hair, you get a great haircut. If you're happy with his work, you have no issues paying him a decent fee for his services. The amount you pay is proportional to how well you think he's done and the value you have in having a great haircut. If you go to a personal trainer, on the other hand, and they give you a great workout, provide you with a diet plan, and are extremely thorough with checking in on you, what happens when you don't get results?

From a business perspective, it's your responsibility to explain to people that lack of compliancy isn't just bad for your business; it's actually a waste of their money. It's due diligence and quality control. It has nothing to do with having an array of 'before and afters' and being known as a transformation coach. If people are giving you their money for no reason year in year out with no change, you shouldn't just take it. Mentally, emotionally, and statistically, deadwood is detrimental to growth. Calculate how much each client returns per unit of time and then Pumpkin Plan your business by putting attention into your clients with the most potential who are happy to invest in you.

BUSINESS PERIODISATION

Breaking Down Phases

You'll be amazed how many times the principles we apply to training can be applied to business. Often, however, we overlook them because they're so glaringly obvious. This section will explain why periodisation isn't just useful in business; it's an essential part of long term growth and maximising your time.

Strength training periodisation was my first love in the fitness industry. As soon as I became fixated on getting as strong as possible, I started to obsess over numbers and rep schemes. It may not surprise you, but I was very analytical about performance and so I read up on every method out there. For those who aren't as programme design savvy, the arrangement of blocks of training is known as periodisation. This is where you periodise working on a specific quality in order to achieve a certain goal. For example, you may spend four weeks working in an 8–12 rep range to build muscle and then four weeks working in a 4–6 rep range to gain strength. There are many types of periodisation. Traditionally you have linear periodisation, where you work from high reps down to low reps in a linear fashion. This is popular among many powerlifting coaches. There is also something called undulating periodisation. This is where you go from one block to another, then back to the initial block but slightly modified. For example, four weeks at 10–12 reps, then four weeks at 4–6 reps, then four weeks at 9–11 reps. Think of it as a wave where the height slowly lowers over time.

I used this method of training for a long time. I gravitated towards it because the goal was to cement a certain quality before moving on to the next phase. You had objectives to reach in each phase that potentiated your development in the proceeding block. So, for four weeks you'd get as strong as possible in the 10–12 reps range before dropping to lower reps. This ensured you have adequate strength/endurance capacity and tendon integrity before handling higher loads. The higher rep scheme phases are known as accumulation phases. This is because volume of reps is the goal and not weight on the bar. When you drop to lower reps, your goal is to handle more weight. This is otherwise known as a higher intensity of your one rep max and is called an intensification phase. After years of utilising this programme structure in the quest to get stronger, I had a sudden realisation when looking to seek business clarity and direction. Why am I not applying this to my business?

You see, you only have so many hours in the day and so many available times to work. Although you can get smaller jobs such as admin and social media posts done in a relatively small amount of time, further development projects do require a lot more focused effort. It's incredibly hard to juggle several jobs at once and if you're not careful, you'll start to notice less work getting done and your session quality slipping. You need to be purposeful with what you're looking to achieve in a designated amount of time and make peace with projects or elements that may need to be put on the back burner.

A game changer for me was when I split my year into quarters. I wrote a business model for every twelve months with a goal of how many sessions I wanted to deliver and how much money I wanted to make. I registered as a limited company at the end of November 2017, meaning my financial year starts in December. Unbeknown to me, this was actually a fortunate move because my financial quarters had fallen on periods of the year that followed certain trends. December, January, and February were typically quiet months for me. Everyone was both physically and financially recovering from Christmas, meaning that both session delivering and PT uptake was lower than average. This changed in March through to May when a lot of people were focusing on getting into beach body condition. If you have an affluent client base, it is likely that they'll go away at some point during the summer holidays. Again, this means both delivery and uptake suffer. This wasn't necessarily the case for June and midway through July, but August notoriously followed the same trend as Christmas. Again, just like the March boom in demand for personal training, the same happened from September through November. Everyone wants to get in the best shape possible before over-indulging during the festive season. I noticed these trends for two years. This made me think, "Why aren't I capitalising on this?"

Have you got an idea that you'd love to bring to fruition? A book you'd love to write? A podcast you want to get up and running? How about building a social media presence so you attract an online clientele? The reality is that these things take time and effort. Worrying about writing the perfect social media post whilst delivering eight sessions a day is only going to add to your stresses. It's not going to contribute positively to your business and it's only going to lead to the feeling of being overwhelmed. Chase two rabbits, catch neither. Each phase, you must differentiate whether your goal is to earn money in the trenches or to build your own content and brand. This will take the pressure off and give objective goals to work to. Let's look at an example.

You're busy. Busy is good and you have a thriving one-to-one personal training business that earns you a respectable amount of money. The problem is that you've been doing this for five years straight now. Getting to the gym for 5:00am and leaving at 9:00pm is starting to take its toll. You'd love to work more flexible hours but are scared what working less would do to your income. Ideally, building an online client base would accommodate for your working schedule desires; however, you've never been able to build an online presence due to working in the gym so much. Any down time is spent either training or unwinding. Situations like this scream out for business model periodisation. So, what do you do?

First, you need to assess your finances. You need to know how much you spend on average each month. This will give you your average outgoings, which is arguably *the* most important factor in this situation. You must be able to fill in the blank in this sentence, "I need £… per month to cover all my outgoings." You need to assess your current client base, who is down to renew, who may drop off, who is going on holiday, and what time of the year it is. Are you going into an accumulation phase (high volume of sessions delivered), or an intensification phase (time where you can work on the business and brand)? Break this phase in to a twelve-week period and set some objective, data-driven goals you can assess.

Example Accumulation Phase

Deliver 334 sessions in the next twelve weeks. As the average session rate is currently £30, this equates to £10,000. Track all outgoings so you're aware of your expenses going into the proceeding phase. Social media posts will be kept to 2–3 posts a week, purely posting about your own training, clients, and food. This will take less than one hour per week. The goal isn't to drive up followers, it's to keep your social media account ticking over. Any gained followers are a bonus. Reading material will be kept to weekends and in the evening if you desire. Your sole focus is to work on in person client satisfaction and ensure that all your clients are extremely happy with your services. You are working *in* your business so that revenue goes up. You quantify your progress by tracking how much you earn and how many sessions you deliver. If this drops, you need to work on getting referrals through your own client base. Given that you are full and couldn't take anybody else on, 4–6 weeks left of an accumulation phase is the perfect time to send out an email increasing your prices.

Example Intensification Phase

This is a period where your goal should be to capitalise on having more time to dedicate towards self-development. You'll be getting quieter and you could even promote a drop off in clientele by increasing your prices. Say you have a client who's been with you for years and never had a price increase. Raising their fees going into an intensification phase would be perfect as they'll either drop off or pay you more. It's a win-win as your goal here is to reduce the amount of time you're working on the gym floor. However, I wouldn't increase prices going into December. Logistically, it makes no sense. If March to May is another accumulation phase, I'd say May/June time is a good time to give 4–6 weeks' notice of a price increase. This means you'll be increasing your prices at this point every year. An annual increase in fees at the same point each year would be wise, unless you are in demand enough to do otherwise.

You still need objective data to assess, therefore your goal is to deliver 250 sessions in the next twelve weeks at an average of £30 per hour. This means you earn £7,500 for that phase. During your intensification phase, you again need objective data to work off. This could be to complete an online training course, set up a podcast and record six sessions to have pre-recorded content, or increase the social media posting frequency so my following goes up by 300 in twelve weeks. You need goals and figures to judge how successful a phase has been. The key thing is that this phase has contributed to giving you the ability to earn more money. You have either educated yourself so that you bring more value to your one-to-one clients and can therefore charge more, or you have developed on online service or product you can sell to people. Just like undulating periodisation, your goal here is to overload over time. You spend two phases a year in your business working incredibly hard and then two phases a year on your business to give you the potential to earn more money during your accumulation phases. If in year 1 your average rate is £30 an hour and you do 330 sessions during an accumulation phase, you'll earn £9,990 in those twelve weeks. If by year 3, your average rate is £40 an hour and you do 330 sessions during an accumulation phase, you'll earn £13,200 in those twelve weeks. That's a 33% increase in revenue by doing the same number of hours. Your brand develops, your reputation develops, and your income develops. You could even use this opportunity to drop your evening hours and work more on your terms, but more on that later.

Still apprehensive? That's fine, but this is why tracking your outgoings is so important. A lot of people are scared to work less and charge more. However, if you think about it, if you know your outgoings to a tee, you should be able to live off your savings. If your total outgoings are £2,000 a month, you need £6,000 to live for the next twelve weeks. If you earn £9,990 during an accumulation phase and are smart with your money, you should have £3,990 remaining. This means that just to get by, you'd need to earn £2,010 in the next twelve weeks to cover all your outgoings. If you charge £30 an hour, this is sixty-seven sessions in the next twelve weeks, working out at six sessions a week. Even if you drop off in session delivery due to time or year and increasing prices, you're extremely unlikely to go this low. An accumulation phase shouldn't just be about earning money for the sake of it. It should be about providing an element of financial freedom so that you are focused on personal development in the next phase. As long as you save and deliver around 15–20 sessions per week, you'll be more than fine to see a drop off in delivery. You just need to ensure you're being astute with your down time and working on and tracking growth.

THE 5 X 5 RULE FOR BUSINESS

Business is highly reliant on objective, measurable data. It requires tracking, assessments, and analysis of the market to validate growth. The following rules are based on these principles and give a precise strategy to utilise in relation to your own goals.

Option 1: Increase fees by 5% or £5, every time five people buy a block of sessions at a certain rate

Option 2: Increase fees by 5% or £5 once a year at the same time each year

Imagine your hourly rate lies on a continuum. Here, £25 an hour is at the lower end of the spectrum, whilst £100 an hour is on the higher end. Your goal is to move yourself along this line the longer you spend in the industry. A 5% increase is a marginal step forward, whereas £5 is a big jump in the right direction. The traditional prices of personal training sessions usually ascend in jumps of £2.50, and you could opt for this increment if you wish as well. The most important thing is that you have a systematic way of measuring and justifying growth. I have chosen 5% as the minimum rate of increase for several reasons. First, it's because it's significant enough to see an improvement in rates over time, but not high enough to encounter a high level of complaint from your clients. If you're working hard to provide the best possible training experience for a client and they're getting results, there should be no resistance in them going from £35 to £36.75 an hour. If you consider the average rate of inflation (currently around 2.1% July 2019), your prices **should** increase by at least 2% per year. The extra 3% accounts for your growing experience, knowledge, and investment in education.

Prior to talking about the 5 x 5 rule, I first laid the foundations of what the rule is about and how you can apply it to your business. Education leads to understanding. The more you understand the benefits of something, the more you're likely to stick to it. Think of it like explaining to your clients about calories and macros. As their knowledge of these factors increase, so does the likely of them sticking to a plan. If they don't get results, they start to understand why. It's all well and good me telling you to put up your rates and work the hours you want but believing it's as simple as that is naive. You may have a model, but you have to have pre-requisites for growth. The principle of the 5 x 5 rule for business works on two different levels: one for the more ambitious trainer and one for the more conservative. For those of you with more lofty goals, the 5 x 5 rule is that once five people have bought a block of sessions for a set price, you increase your rates by either 5% or £5, whichever you see as more appropriate. If doing this doesn't seem feasible to you just yet, go with the second option of increasing your fees by 5% at the same time on an annual basis. Let's look at an example.

Say you charge £360 for a block of twelve sessions. This works out at £30 an hour. You are currently training twelve clients working out at twenty-four sessions per week on average. If you want to earn more money, your choices are either to take on more clients or increase fees. If you want to earn a lot more money, you should do both. The problem is, working more is a slippery slope. You're doing early starts, late nights, your training suffers, and so does your social life.

Session delivery to working week can have anything from a 25–50% increase in the personal training world. It all depends how good you are with your time. What I mean by this is that if you deliver thirty sessions, your working week is anywhere from 38–45 hours. It's rare to fit people in back to back consistently, so you'll end up spending a lot of time at work by default. This is why for me, an ideal session delivery for most personal trainers is twenty-five a week. This way you still shouldn't be working any more than forty hours a week, which is the going norm. I spoke earlier about managing finances and figuring out the minimum amount of time you need to work to get by. To figure this out, you divide your average monthly outgoings by your current hourly rate. Let's say £2,000/30 in this case. This would mean that after delivering sixty seven sessions, everything else is profit. A hundred sessions per month means that thirty-three sessions account for savings and non-essential expenses. By now you should be aware that these are kept to a minimum.

If you're saving up for a house, wedding, or holiday, it's easy to say yes to people and load up your diary, especially if you're in demand. The problem is that this is the path of least resistance and it'll build a poor outlook on your work to earnings ratio. You'll start to believe that the less you work, the less you get paid. This shouldn't be the case. You have to be able to say no to people; you have to be able to turn down money if earning it isn't on your terms. Money is important, but it's just one component of happiness. What's the point in having a large bank account if you never see your family, are in a gym sixteen hours a day, and can't even train yourself? My point is, unless you're saving for a specific target, you shouldn't aim to deliver as many sessions as humanly possible. This isn't being work shy; it's smart time management. It means you can build other revenues of income such as an online training brand, but most importantly, have a good work life balance and get to see your family. Personal trainers love to go on about how many sessions they do. It's like you earn some sort of badge of honour by saying you've done 40–50 sessions a week. The most I've ever done for a sustained period is around the

35–40 mark. All it taught me is that the more I worked, the worse my delivery got and the less amount of time I had to dedicate towards growth. If someone said to me now that they do over forty sessions a week, I wouldn't be impressed, I'd be confused as to why they haven't increased their rates if they're in such high demand. I'm going to reiterate the point so it sinks in: unless you are specifically saving for an event that requires more funds than usual, why are you working at the expense of your health and wellbeing? I believe that twenty-five sessions a week is the sweet spot for a personal trainer. However, if we take into account the undulating periodisation model of business, this may look like twenty sessions per week in one phase and thirty in another. It's important that you identify a capacity per phase.

Once you are consistently doing thirty hours per week during an accumulation phase, you are full. If you're not doing this amount, your goal is to get to this point charging a rate you feel comfortable with and so therefore have no problem loading up your diary. The golden rule of the 5 x 5 model is that price increases are only warranted when demand exceeds supply. In other words, you need to be busy. If you're not busy, price increases must wait. If you're wondering on how to get busy, revisit the lead generation section and ensure you're doing everything it says on a daily basis.

If you reach capacity during a training phase and are getting new inquiries for personal training, you should quote the new inquiry for 5% or £5 more than your current hourly rate. This is because demand has exceeded supply and your popularity is testament to the fact that you need to charge more. If you are going into an accumulation phase where session delivery is going to be high and you are still getting more inquiries, this means you would exceed capacity. In this scenario, prices should go up by 5% for existing clients who have not experienced a price increase for over a year. However, as I mentioned before, a price increase going into December would be extremely unwise. You are making people spend more money with you at a time where their expenses will be the highest.

If putting up an existing client's rate scares you, don't worry; I had the same apprehensions. It's completely natural but is a limiting mindset when it comes to growth. First things first: people wouldn't train with you for years if you weren't good at what you do. If this is the case, they should respect you enough to realise that you deserve a small and justified pay rise for your efforts. Second, how much effort and energy have you put into your education and development for these people? Are you the same trainer who was training them two years ago? What have you learned in that time? You need to recuperate your investments into education and it should come from your clients. The moment you detach yourself from the notion that asking for more money is a negative trait, your business will grow exponentially. You cannot fear rejection. If people cannot afford you, it's not your problem. It's your mission to make sure you're a necessity, not nicety. Another thing that cannot go unmentioned is the inflation in the cost of living per year. House prices, petrol, commuting fees, even basic groceries all undergo inflation rates. Therefore, each year you deliver the same amount of monthly sessions and don't increase your rates, you're losing money. This is why so many trainers opt to work more over improving their business and developing.

A 5% inflation rate means your £360 for twelve sessions would increase to £378. It's minimal but all adds up. I honestly think most people can stretch an extra £18 in their budget, especially for such a useful commodity. The good thing about this is that it's periodic. If you explain to your loyal client base that you review your rates every six months, increases will be normal to them. In one year, you go from £30 an hour to £33 an hour. Doesn't seem like much, but at a twenty-five sessions a week, that's an extra £300/month and £3,600/year. Would you say no to an extra £3,600 just to prevent having an awkward conversation with a client? I want you to realise that this is business and if you present yourself in the right way, are professional in your manner, and give your clients excellent value, they will understand. Most of them will be businesspeople too, after all.

Once you build confidence in your own ability, plus have the safety net of a loyal client base to provide a steady income, your goal should be to increase your hourly rate for new inquiries. If an inquiry says no due to price, you are no worse off than you were before; if they say yes, you have a new higher paying client. It also means that if you increase your rates for existing clients and they don't like it, you can replace them with a higher paying client. It may sound ruthless but it's business. If you are good at what you do and don't have this approach, you are short-changing yourself. One hurdle you may face with this method is if your new inquiry comes via word of mouth from an existing client. They may expect to get the sessions at the same rate as their friend and could even be offended if you charge them more. This is why it is essential to review your rates on a regular basis and always assess your hourly rate. Remember, you are only worth what your lowest hourly rate is paying you. If you have new clients who are paying £50 and ones who have been with you for years paying £30, you are still a £30 an hour trainer. At any given point, a client could refer someone to you. Therefore, it is essential that you review everyone's fees and look to periodically increase them by a valid margin. When I first went self-employed in 2013, my average rate was £25 an hour. From 2014 to 2018, some of my clients saw their hourly rate double in price. I've had some people stay and some people drop off, but they've always been replaced by new clients paying the new rate.

To make things a little clearer, think of things like this. Say you own a shoe shop that sells designer trainers. Due to the size of your shop, you only have space for a hundred pairs of shoes in stock. You have a pair of trainers in the window that make you a £25 profit per sale. They're popular and sell out each month with every order you put in. You also have a pair of trainers that make you £10 profit per sale. They're not as popular and don't sell out each month. You initially used to buy fifty pairs of each shoe, but after reviewing your sales over the past months, you start to re-think this idea. When your sales rep comes in and asks how much of each shoe you want, which ones do you order and in what quantity?

This analogy may seem painfully straight forward. You'd obviously want to order more of the profitable shoe, right? Even someone with limited business experience could see this. Why would you stock a shoe that takes up space when you could have a more profitable option available? Hopefully you can see where I'm going with this.

The only difference between this analogy and your business is that one is dealing with the inanimate objects of footwear and the other is people with whom you've built rapport. You can't hurt a shoe's feelings, but it is possible to offend a long-term client whose rates haven't been adjusted in five years. This is why assessment of growth and periodic increases are essential in business. Whether there is any resistance will boil down to your client's perception of value in you and your own perception of value in yourself. Therefore, it's a necessity to constantly work on both. The people who are paying you the same rates they were on several years ago are like the less profitable shoe. They are taking up space where you could be earning more money. Now I understand that you'll have built a relationship with them, but this is where you've blurred the lines between socialising and business. It's the most common mistake in personal training. You can and should build rapport with your clients, but it must be done in a manner where they see the integrity and formality in your business. This is your work and you should treat it like that.

Getting used to the price increasing process is difficult. It's a scary step but one you know yourself needs to be taken. Please remember though, I'm not hell bent on you increasing your fees because I'm some business mogul who's fixated on wealth. I just want you to gain the confidence to ask for the money you deserve. As discussed earlier, £30 an hour doesn't always go a long way. There are a lot of trainers out there under charging purely through a lack of confidence and belief. Once this barrier is broken, it becomes a natural process that gets easier each time you do it. This is why I recommend increasing your rates by £5 or 5% for existing clients, given that you are hitting your delivery quotation. It will give you more money to invest into education, more time to spend developing your brand, and less pressure to work every hour God sends to earn ends meet. If you want to be in this game for the long run and build a product you're proud of, you have to get outside your comfort zone when it comes to business.

I believe that any personal trainer should be able to make £60,000 a year gross income by the end of the fifth year of their business model. That is obviously a monumental statement given that the average annual salary in the UK is around £30,000 (stated in 2019) and the average earnings of a personal trainer is estimated to be £20,000 per year. Sound far-fetched? Consider this.

Say a personal trainer gets qualified and starts out in a commercial gym. They don't pay rent but charge £40 per hour a session, to which they get paid £15 an hour. By month six of their business they build up to consistently delivering fifteen sessions per week on average. They are also doing sixteen hours of gym shifts a week on £7.50 per hour. Their theoretical annual earnings (TAE) would be £15,525 based on a forty-eight week year (to which all calculations are based). By month twelve of their business they are doing twenty sessions a week and eight hours on the gym floor (TAE: £20,160). They then realise that they have reached their earning capacity in a commercial gym setting and so opt to move gyms to either another commercial gym or independent facility with a rent-based option. This increases their outgoings but improves their earning potential. They make the move and some clients follow. As a way of retaining clients they drop their rates to £30 an hour (an 100% increase in what they take home per hour). By month eighteen of the model, they again average fifteen hours a week but this time earning £30 an hour (TAE: £21,600). If by month twenty-four they increase their average hourly rate by 5% and increase to session delivery to twenty per week, they are now at a TAE of £30,240. This is equal to the average UK salary; however, you have to consider that this PT could be paying anywhere between £500–800 in gym rent per year, meaning that net profit before their personal expenses is going to be around £22,500. I don't want to pull the wool over anyone's eyes here. I am talking £60,000 in earnings and not accounting for outgoings in this example.

In year 3 the trainer has a different focus. They want to educate themselves and build an online brand. They focus purely on development and consistently putting out content online. In this time they use the 5 x 5 model and consistently deliver twenty-five sessions per week whilst making the annual increase of 5%. TAE is now £39,690 by the end of year 3. Month 36–42 is an aggressive accumulation phase for the trainer. They average thirty sessions a week but with a set objective, they want to earn enough money so that they can save to be able to change their working and increase their fees for new client by £5 per hour. They also want to capitalise on their growing online presence by venturing into the world of online coaching. Due to the popularity of their services, they increase their current clients' hourly rate from £33 to £35 and new inquiries to £40. It leads to a drop in session uptake from an average of thirty sessions to twenty sessions; however, this was accounted for in the business model. The goal of month 43–48 is to acquire five online clients paying £75 a month for online coaching. If the trainer is now doing twenty sessions a week on an average of £37.50 an hour with five online clients paying £75 per month, the TAE is £40,500. It's a modest increase by the end of year 4 but some excellent foundations have been set. If in the next twelve months the trainer increases their online client base by one client per month, whilst simultaneously driving session delivery up to twenty-five sessions per week, TAE will be £60,300. They will be earning double the average annual wage whilst delivering five sessions a day, when they desire, and not working weekends. This is based on logical, planned progressions taking into consideration quality of service, validating fees, and a sound business model. You have a plan and you stick to it. There will obviously be an element of variance in your earnings, but this can be in both a positive and negative way. Although client uptake may be lower than anticipated, you may choose to charge more than £37.50 an hour and £75 a month for online. It goes without saying you hit your £60,000 a year target much quicker if you charge more (given that you're busy). To make things extremely simple, if you're charging £40 an hour per one-to-one session and £100 a month online by year 5 of your business, twenty-five sessions per week and ten online clients creates £60,000 gross revenue over the period of a forty-eight-week year.

Now, it's important to note that this is gross revenue. In your five years you may meet your partner, have a family, look to buy a house, and so forth. Earning £5,000 per month may sound incredible, but the likelihood is your outgoings will rise too. I would estimate that once tax, gym rent, plus regular personal and business outgoings are accounted for, your net profit will be around ~£1,500 per month. That's still £18,000 a year to play with, which you can't complain about. My point is, I don't want to deceive you. I want you to earn more so you get to stay in this game for the long run whilst working the hours you want without sacrificing your health. Why? Because the more well-educated, high-quality, and well-paid personal trainers there are out there, the more we stand of making a lasting positive change on the health of a generation. We as trainers need to earn more so that we can be better at what we do. What I find exciting is the possibilities of what can happen if you continue to use this model for another five years. This all depends on the rate of your development, which leads to the question, what do we need to do in order to develop?

Now that you have a model, you need to fill in the gaps. We established the figures that need to be achieved month to month, but how do we grow in this time? How do we attract new clients, get busy, increase fees, and build an online brand? In part two of the book, we'll address you the person—your daily habits, education, and productivity—to you the brand—your content, your ethos, and your ability to create fans who want to work with you. This is my guide to enhancing all of what I consider the essentials of a personal trainer's arsenal in order to develop at a rate sequential to your business plan.

SELF DEVELOPMENT

THE REALITY OF SELF DEVELOPMENT

We are not the result of what we do; we are the result of what we do consistently. I'm sure anyone reading this has their good days, the ones where everything goes to plan and you feel like you've gotten a lot done. It's a great feeling. My goal for you is to consolidate that satisfaction and make it into a daily occurrence. Procrastination is the thief of progression. If we don't set up our diary and create habits that positively contribute to our growth and development, no amount of motivation will prove effective. There's not a great deal of difference between you growing your business and your client losing weight. It all boils down to your habits and what you find the easiest to sustain.

I need you to sit down for an hour a day and write a thousand words. It doesn't matter whether you're tired or not in the right frame of mind to work, just sit down and don't do anything else until a thousand words are written. This is how you grow your business—just kidding. I had you for a second there, didn't I? Forcing yourself to work is a lot like forcing a client to eat a carrot stick when they've been used to enjoying a chocolate bar on their lunch break. You're relying too much on will power and that is a finite commodity that decreases under stress. The more hectic your life gets, the less likely you are to do the things that require the most energy and discipline. This happens to everyone, so don't be harsh on yourself when productivity waivers under testing times. I meditate, stretch, diaphragmatically breathe, eat well, write, express gratitude, and write out my goals on a daily basis. These are all components that we'll be discussing in this section.

There are days when I don't do these things. Work stress, poor sleep, deadlines, and family commitments can mean these things get pushed to the side. Although in an ideal world they'd get done, sometimes they don't, and that's okay. I think we as PTs are guilty of wanting to be perfect. We want to be seen as robots who are incredibly regimented and work every hour God sends in order to reach our potential. If we're not working, we're slacking. I had this mindset for a long time. I couldn't switch off. Even if it was 9:00pm and I'd done all the tasks I needed to do that day, I'd then get out an anatomy book and start studying. Part of the reason came from wanting to learn, but the majority of it was so I felt like I was doing something productive. Actions aren't necessarily productive, results are. You can take a lot of action and not get any results, whereas if you're precise, focused, and efficient, results will come as a by-product of well executed habits.

Before we begin the self-development section, I first want you to make peace with the fact that you'll never be the finished article. Self-development is on-going and no one who achieved excellency in any domain ever turned around and said, "Yeah, I'm done now." The wise know that you can never stop learning and developing. Your goal after reading this book is to create realistic, sustainable habits that lead to objectively measured growth. You will gain the ability to assess your diary, see what needs focus, see when you can focus on it, and create a day with the greatest likelihood of achieving success. Work with yourself, not against yourself. There's no point in planning to do five client programmes in a thirty-minute gap between sessions when you're more likely to chat to peers. You've got to be realistic. Sitting down in a coffee shop and brain dumping 1,500 words of content is awesome. However, it's not awesome if it's done once every two weeks during a moment of highly caffeinated inspiration. Writing 250 words a day, on the other hand, can be done in thirty minutes. If you do this five days a week for two weeks, you'll have 2,500 words in the same amount of time. This is measurable, objective content that can help develop your brand and service. This is what you need to focus on. Brick by brick, one step at a time, your goal is to create momentum and put energy into what yields the greatest rewards.

CHANGING YOUR PRODUCTIVITY MINDSET

As you may have noticed, I liken business development to weight loss several times in this book. The reason for this is that success rates have universal laws. It's about habit formation, mindset, and environment. If you had a client who ate their lunch in a cafeteria where all their colleagues were eating burgers, pizza, and cakes, they're not in the best environment to create lifelong change. If the client got into the routine of going for a walk, finding a park bench, and enjoying a chicken wrap and salad, they'd have much better foundations for getting results. What's the biggest obstruction in your current development and how do you change it?

The first thing you must do is to begin each day with an action plan. A plan creates tasks and a day's productivity levels can be assessed by how many of these tasks you get done. I recommend beginning each day with five minutes of meditation (or deep breathing if you're not sure how to meditate) and then write down all the things that must be done that day. Don't begin with the things you'd like to do; begin with the things that must be done for your business to grow. Begin your meditation or breathing by first scanning the body. Bring awareness to your breath and focus on 3D expansion of the mid-section. Breathe in through the nose for four seconds, then out through the nose for four seconds. Calm your body, calm your thoughts, and lock yourself in. Once you have quietened down your mind, start to focus on all the things you are grateful for in your life. Think about what makes you happy. Think about the people you love. Think about how your body reacts and feels when spending time with a loved one. Recreate these emotions whilst maintaining your rhythmic breathing. Once you have done this, start to think about your day. Think about how you can carry these positive emotions and pass them on to other people. How can you make your clients and colleagues feel better about themselves? How can you provide so much value that people are grateful to be working with you? What do these actions entail and look like? Once you have created a clear picture of what you need to do, gently bring your meditation to an end, pick up a pen, and write.

Have you ever watched one of those psychological horror films where the villain is created in your own imagination? They're always lurking in the shadows or under the bed with sinister intent. You never see what the monster looks like, but it petrifies you because there's incredible tension and fear surrounding their presence. This is similar to what it's like when you feel overwhelmed but don't write down a to-do list. You feel scared about the mammoth tasks you must do, but because you don't write them down and physically see them, the fears grow and seem ever more intimidating. It's not until you see your work list that you realise it's a lot more manageable than you thought. Personally, I love *The High Performance Planner* designed by Brendon Burchard. If you type it in on Amazon, it's the black book available in three-, six-, and twelve-month packages. It accompanies this morning routine perfectly as you can then write up your day with clarity. You need to ask yourself, "What are the most important things I need to do to grow my business and at what part of the day am I most likely to do them?"

If you've ever felt overwhelmed, stressed out by work, and feel you've bitten off more than you can chew, simply write down a list of every single thing you have to do. Don't leave anything off the list, write down absolutely everything you can think of. Then give each task a rating from one to three. One is for tasks that need to be done today without fail, two is for tasks that need to be done this week, and three is for long-term projects that can be done when you have some spare time. It's likely the number one ranked tasks are the ones you've been putting off for a while and now need completing ASAP, like the client programmes and diet plans you still haven't managed to get around to. I call these "the tasks of most resistance" and its essential that you get these completed as early as possible in your day. If we revisit the notion of will power, you'll recall that I said it was a finite commodity that you deplete. Whether this is scientifically true I have no idea, but the way I see it we become less likely to do more demanding tasks the further we get into our day. Stress, tiredness, and distraction become more present. The urgency we had to do a task turns in to "I'll do it tomorrow." This attitude probably led you to getting overwhelmed in the first place. What you'll find if you address your "tasks of most resistance" as early as possible is that your feelings of helplessness quickly diminish and are replaced with ones of satisfied productivity.

One of the ways I managed to get a lot done was by writing a list each day and doing the things I didn't want to do first. I put the most amount of importance on these tasks and knew that getting them out the way would lead to huge relief. To do this, I changed my mindset towards what I had to do and instead would dangle a proverbial carrot for myself to get the job done quicker. For example, I love writing. I'd happily sit down and write parts of my book or social media posts at any time of the day. As a coach, I have to write a high volume of diet and training plans. It's not that I don't like doing these things, but they do take time, patience, and thoroughness, especially if I'm calculating someone's macros per meal gram for gram. These are the things that I will put off the most. I'll jovially write thousands of words that contribute to a greater project, but this distracts from more immediately important jobs that are a necessity to maintain the quality of my business. I was prioritising a number three task over a number one task.

This led me to getting stressed, even more so when a client texted or emailed to say, "Any luck with the diet plan?" I hate that, mainly because it's highlighting my own lack of organisation.

You've got to look at it like this. Say you're about to do a workout you've done before. You love the workout as it has Romanian deadlifts in it. You're good at Romanian deadlifts and can shift a lot of weight. The only problem is, you have to do rack-supported Bulgarian split squats before the deadlifts and these are horrible. You absolutely hate them. You hate the burn, the setup, the rep range. Even though it's just a couple of sets, you dread the thought of having to do them. However, your coach has put them in your programme as your quads need work and were identified as a weak point. Would you skip them? Of course not. If you did, you'd be cheating yourself, you'd be making your life easy, and you wouldn't be committed to holistic self-improvement. Just like there are exercises in your programme you don't relish doing, there are tasks in your day that need to be completed.

How do you change your mindset to turn arduous tasks in to ones that you enjoy? By seeing the bigger picture. Working on weaknesses leads to greater growth. Just like bringing up a lagging body part improves the appearance of your entire physique, completing the tasks you struggle with most will help your overall productivity levels. You don't *have* to do the tasks on your list, you *get* to do them. By completing the tricky tasks early on, you create more time to do the ones that you like. Therefore, doing the tasks of most resistance as soon as possible makes a lot of sense. You are freeing up more time for enjoyable tasks during the day. Don't ever run away from discomfort. Tackle it head on and address it immediately. If you do this with your day, you'll not only get more work done, you'll free up your time for more enjoyable tasks and self-development. If you procrastinate because you don't want to face the tasks you've been putting off, nothing gets done. This is when your workload mounts and you get that feeling of being overwhelmed.

Client's cancelling can be frustrating. It can mess up your day and make you feel like you've lost momentum. I used to get annoyed when clients cancelled but then I realised something extremely useful; I'd been granted bonus time. Say you wake up and make your list. You have two client programmes and a diet plan to design, 250 words to write for your website, and an entire module of your online nutrition course to study. You have five clients booked in that day between 6–9am and 4–6pm. During the day you need to eat, train, eat again, and find time to complete your to-do list. Now there are already five hours out of your day dedicated to training people. You won't be able to do any of your tasks during this time, so this is where you are solely working in your business. However, if a client cancels you have just been granted a totally free hour you weren't expecting. See this as a gift of time. The second you know the client isn't turning up, take your things, find a place to work, and complete the one task you least want to do that day. Don't do anything else other than that task. Set your phone to airplane mode, find a quiet place with no distractions, and focus. Getting into the habit of doing this will do wonders for your productivity, workload management, and most of all, happiness and clarity.

ELIMINATING DISTRACTIONS

Do you procrastinate a lot? Does one check of your phone turn into five minutes of mindless scrolling? Do you struggle to start and finish projects? This section will talk you through how to set up the best environment for productivity and create the best chances of getting your tasks done.

Have you ever seen that experiment when they put jellybeans in front of five-year-olds and tell them not to eat them? They tell the five-year-old that if they don't eat the sweet, they'll receive another jellybean when the adult returns. Quite a few of the children complete the task, but they're absolutely encapsulated by the candy in the process. Some smell it, some play with it, some even lick it and place it on their tongue. The jellybean is there, so this is all they can put their focus into. The reward to double the candy is not as intoxicating as having the sweet now because it is at the forefront of their attention. Kids, hey? So young, so naive; I bet you wouldn't find it anywhere near as hard to say no to one measly jellybean for five minutes. Or would you? You'd be surprised that even as adults how much we revert to our inner child. We're not that different from children, we just get preoccupied with more consuming tasks.

Let's use the jellybean experiment as an analogy. You are the child, the jellybean is your phone, and the extra jellybean is the task you need to complete. I believe that when an activity involves a high reward response (big hit of dopamine), future consequences are put to the wayside. So, in Lehman's terms, if it involves sex, food or survival, what happens now is much more important than what might happen in the future. Got a weigh in on Monday but have a piece of double chocolate fudge cake in front of you after your Sunday dinner? Suddenly the weigh in doesn't seem so important. The problem is, food, sex, and survival—the important stuff—are being replaced by totally irrelevant information such as social media content and instant hits of dopamine. This isn't because your brain is searching for pleasure; it's because it's anticipating it. The chase is always better than the catch. I don't actually view things this way, but the primal brain does. It's proposed that there's a bigger increase in dopamine upon the anticipation of a pleasurable event than there is during the actual event itself. You don't go on your phone because you're actively looking for entertainment, but because you might find something entertaining. There's a difference and it plays a big role in productivity. Will power is not the best way to avoid distraction. Keep saying this to yourself and use it as a mantra when looking to get a task done. Task completion is dependent on the environment you set yourself up in and the habits you create. Will power is relatively useless. It's not that you are weak if you get distracted when trying to focus; it's that your brain is actually designed to be distracted by things.

I listened to a fantastic book on Audible called *Atomic Habits* by James Clear. He spoke about similar principles and I was pleased to learn I was already doing a lot of the things he mentions in the book. If productivity really interests you, I couldn't recommend his book enough. He's a huge advocate of setting up the correct environment for work and how it potentiates productivity. The initial draft of this book was over 100,000 words. Sounds like a lot, doesn't it? You may either think, "Wow, he really knows how to get work done," or more likely, "He must really have a lot of time on his hands." The truth is, it's a bit of both. I'd estimate that I wrote 80–90% of the content of this book whilst sat on the train. The train has no WiFi and so I can't stop to scroll through social media or search the internet for any other random stuff I don't need. All distractions were pretty much removed. If I'm posting online, I upload the post between when I get on and the first stop. I then put my phone in my bag and don't check it (for anything) until the penultimate stop. This gives me approximately forty-five minutes to write, completely distraction-free, on my laptop. This, I believe, is when the magic happens. If you have distractions at your disposal, they will always impede your productivity. You will be the child sniffing, smelling, and touching the candy until the temptation becomes too intense. How many times do you say to yourself, "I just can't get in the zone"? It's got nothing do to with inspiration or being focused; it's all about the cues and habits that are stopping you from concentrating in the first place. Here are the best ways to create an ideal working environment.

1. Your phone is not on your person or is in another room.
2. You turn off the WiFi on your laptop.
3. If you need the internet, you use an app that blocks social media on your laptop. There are many available.
4. Sit in the same place, in the same location, like the same chair in the office.
5. Do not cross-contaminate your workspace. This one is directly from *Atomic Habits*. It pretty much means don't do anything in your precious workspace apart from the job you want to do—so no eating or phone browsing.
6. Use headphones to listen to focusing music. My favourite is binaural beats.
7. Don't leave your place or do anything else until you've hit a quota for the day, like 500 words, one client programme, one muscle learned, or until you need to resume training people again.
8. Rinse and repeat this habit until it becomes automatic.

9. Create a checklist or calendar that you can use to cross off each day you complete your habit. It needs to be a visual reminder that you have created a streak.
10. Have a bigger picture in mind. By doing this I am freeing up more time to work on other projects, finish work earlier, spend more time with my family, or have less to worry about.

What Should You Be Focusing On?

There's a running theme in this book that you may have noticed already: data is king. If you can extrapolate figures from your business and assess them, you have valuable information that can assist with growth. In this case, how do you quantify productivity? There's a difference between feeling focused and getting results. We're now going to look at how you differentiate the two of them.

The *High-Performance Planner* requires you to fill it out in both the morning and evening. This is ideal as you get to review how successful the day has been. If you have five tasks that you needed to get done that day and you only completed four, this would give you an 80% success rate. It's not exact science, as some tasks may bare more relevance than others, but what I like about it is that you can calculate a weekly average and then assess how much work you've actually done. More importantly, you'll be able to see how efficient you're being with your time and whether you're taking steps to scale your business.

This leads us to an essential part of productivity: is what you're working on actually contributing to growth? Say you had a productive week. You had a 90% task completion rate and overall you feel like you managed your time well and got a lot of work done. What other bit of information could you cross reference this with to see if you're on the right track? Would it be followers online from setting time aside to write great social media posts? How about a library of articles you've pre-written for your website to boost activity? What about the number of templates you've designed so programming becomes a lot more manageable? These are useful but not essential. Ultimately, productivity rates need to be correlated to income. Task completion doesn't pay your bills, money does and if your actions aren't contributing to an increase in earnings, you need to reassess how you spend your time. I honestly don't think they'll be many people out there more guilty of this than me. I used to spend a ton of time writing, creating videos, and studying in the quest to be better. The problem was, I was getting frustrated with financial stressors because my income wasn't improving. Self-development is important but it can't come at the expense of earning money—not initially anyway. You need to identify how you generate income and be productive in maximising that. This is what productivity ultimately is: the completion of tasks that make your life easier for yourself.

If you were to begin your day by writing clear and precise tasks, you then have a list to complete. You can track the success rate of your productivity each evening by giving yourself a score or percentage of what you got done, e.g. 80% or 4/5. This will then give you a weekly average if you record it each day. This means that when you assess your earnings for the week, you can also cross reference it against your productivity and see how they contribute to one another. If you see a positive correlation between earnings and productivity, you know you are on the right track. However, just as importantly, you may realise that what you assume to be important isn't contributing to your growth as much as you think. For example, you may want to study for an hour a day and therefore list it as a priority. However, if this gets in the way of marketing or brand development, you're not actually going to have the clientele to use the information you've been studying on. You're working on a secondary importance task at the expense of a primary importance task. It's an easy mistake to make in the world of personal training. You feel like you've gotten a lot done, but unfortunately, it hasn't contributed to anything specific.

If you see a positive correlation between productivity and earnings, then this is an indication you are on the right track and need to continue as you are doing. However, if productivity goes up but income fails to do so or even reduces, you now know you're putting emphasis on the wrong things. Let's look at an example. Say you're a PT who has a relatively small social media following. You have a successful one-to-one business and regularly do over twenty-five sessions per week. You decide you want to improve your productivity and so read up on some physiology and spend an hour a day designing some cool infographics for your social media page. You get a decent response and in the course of a month see you followers increase from 250 to 300. Now, you could view this as a positive; having more followers is never bad thing, right? However, I would argue that you've actually robbed yourself of time that could have been spent maximising an area that makes you money. If you're busy in person and all your customers came from word of mouth, I would say that your main goal would be to increase demand for your one-to-one services so that you can warrant putting up your rates.

As I said in the business section, as soon as demand exceeds supply, increase your fees. You could do this by giving talks, presentations, and networking events at local businesses or at the offices of your most loyal clients. They'll always be willing for you to help the productivity of their own work force. You make money from in person clients, so you need to maximise the lead generation of in person clients. Other avenues may seem important, but in reality, they're just distractions. Focus on what makes you money and put all your energy into that. That's the definition of true productivity in my eyes.

Conversely, this situation does become different if said coach has another agenda. Say you're comfortably doing over twenty-five sessions per week but want to build an online business to supplement your income. Now time invested into social media becomes relevant. As this is the main source where you're likely to generate leads, increasing followers would be a smart plan of action. In this situation, seeing the wood through the trees and being astute with your finances is essential. You need to give yourself the best chance of success without sacrificing the quality of your in-person services.

This is where business periodisation comes in. For systemic growth in multiple areas, you must understand that there will be periods when you must prioritise certain components over others. This must be done whilst simultaneously maintaining the quality of your existing products. If you don't do this, you risk seeing a drop-off in clientele, leading to reduced income. All commitment to self-development must be put on hold the second that your services come into question. If you haven't mastered your *in* business skills, *on* business skills have to wait. Nail the basics first: happy customers.

Campaigns are important as a personal trainer. Going through phases where you put your foot on the gas in one area whilst coasting in another is a key component of having a multifaceted business. Spinning plates is tricky and to get another plate up and running, you first need to ensure that the other plates are spinning self-sufficiently. The tasks that you prioritise must specifically reflect your goals over a given period. If your goal is to get more online clients through social media, focus on social media. If you want to get busier in a one-to-one setting, look to do more face-to-face interactions where people can connect and build rapport with you. If your daily tasks don't complement your business goals, you get busy doing nothing. Productivity becomes irrelevant. You may finish each day with a 100% completion rate, but this isn't reflected by your bank balance. Daily goals need to be specific and specificity lies in what you're looking to achieve during a business phase.

To summarise, there is a big difference between productivity and being busy. Busy is just filling your day with tasks, whereas productivity is an action plan that contributes to the growth or running of your business. It's easy to be busy, but this is usually met with working ungodly hours and feeling overwhelmed. I know when I'm being efficient with my time when I stop working. If it gets to 6:00pm and I've done everything that has to be done that day, I close my laptop, turn off my phone, and stop working. Why? Because anything done past this point is eating into my down time, which potentiates my ability to work when I'm at my best. You shouldn't be working all the time. In fact, if you are, it's a clear sign that you're not being productive.

CONTENT DEVELOPMENT

In the previous chapter I spoke about maximising time and writing out your most important tasks for the day. I'd now like to discuss two aspects I believe are key to a personal trainer's development. Some trainers may feel overwhelmed with workload and the pressure of a thriving business but for others, they may not know where to begin. If this is you, there are certain habits I would highly recommend when it comes to building your PT business. The main two are:

- Spend 10–15 minutes a day learning one muscle
- Spend 20–30 minutes a day writing

Total time: 45 minutes

The reason I recommend learning one muscle a day is that anatomy will always be your saving grace when it comes to training people. The better your anatomy knowledge is, the better trainer you can become. Knowing muscle origins and insertion points will help you when looking to overcome problems caused by structural limitations. Never look to learn more than one muscle a day and don't do anything else until you've made sure you've learnt the muscle properly. Don't be afraid to think outside the box and use alternative methods of remembering things. Imagine an icy cold bottle of Peroni touching the side of your calf. The cold, wet glass giving you a chill that goes up your entire leg. Random? Not quite, the muscles on the side of your calf are called the peroneals. There are three of them: longus, brevus, and tertius. They originate on the lateral superior aspects of the fibula bone and insert between the medial cuniform and metatarsal bones in the feet. Their role is to assist in pronation of the foot and guide external rotation of the knee. Hand on heart, I didn't have to Google that. Taking a little bit of time to learn something in an unconventional way can put an imprint on your brain. Ten minutes' investment into anatomy will make a huge difference in the long run.

What about writing though? Why is writing so important?

Before I begin, I want you to understand something called the flower pot theory of brain capability. It was once thought that our brains were like filing cabinets. They had the capacity to store a lot of info but once all the storage was taken up, it was not possible to take in any more information. This isn't the case. You brain is more like a flower. The more you water it, the more it grows. The only limitation in the ability to grow is the environment and nourishment you give it. My point is, if you do something regularly and do it in a good, nourishing environment, it flows. I wrote 100,000 words for this book purely by writing for forty-five minutes a day, five days a week. Writing content is invaluable because it indicates one thing: dedication. It takes about five minutes to upload a topless selfie, and well written, thorough articles take substantially longer. In this business, you always have to think, how can I stand out and how can I maintain the highest level of integrity? By writing content for your clientele, you are showing them that you care, that you can manage your time well, that you are well read, and that you really want them to get results.

For example, say you have thirty minutes a day before you train. It's when you usually have your pre-workout coffee and will sit and do programmes, read, or go on social media. It's a ritual that you enjoy and have gotten into the habit of. What if you were to replace this habit with one that contributes to your business' growth by instead spending 15–20 minutes writing the answer to and FAQ you get from your one-to-one or online clients. Now, contrary to what people may think, re-writing a textbook on protein consumption and secondary active transport of glucose ingestion is not what your clients want to read about. You'll lose people quick if you try to sound too smart. Remember, people read Cosmo and the Daily Mail for a reason. It's a light, enjoyable read, written in a tone they can relate to. For me, I believe the best blend is one that is semi-educational but anecdotal as well. This is because you're getting information but seeing how it works in the real world.

You've just done three clients back to back from 6:30 to 9:30am. It's 10:30 now. You've eaten and are having your pre-workout coffee before training at noon. During your morning sessions, one of your clients was explaining that they couldn't stick to the diet plan you gave them because Tesco had run out of cod and you'd put it in the diet plan. This is absolutely perfect, as it then allows you to write an article on protein intake for real world people. It may look a little like this.

In your diet plans you will see a certain amount of meat accompanied by the number of grams of it you should eat, e.g. 150 g chicken. Chicken has around 30 g of protein per 100 g, therefore a 150 g portion of raw chicken will provide around 45 g protein once cooked. You need to be eating at least 2 g protein per kilo of body weight. This is to ensure you recover from training properly and can build muscle.

Now in this situation, it is the protein that is important, not necessarily the meat source. You could opt for cod, sea bass, hake, turkey, scampi, prawns, and so on. Switch your meats up so you don't get bored. What I would like you to do, though, is pick a meat that has at least 25 g of protein per 100 g of weight. You can easily find this out by reading the back of the packet.

One thing to keep an eye out for though is fat content. Fat is great but needs to be kept at bay to control calories. If fat is too high, your calorie intake may creep up and you might not see the changes in weight and body composition that you're after. When selecting a meat, make sure the protein is over 25 g per 100 g and the fat content is under 5 g per 100 g.

There you go. You have just diffused a FAQ you're likely to get from most clients who start a fresh with you. It's clear, to the point, didn't have to use any jargon, and tells them what to do in a nutshell. This is just one example of literally thousands of different questions you will and have been asked from your client base. "Do things today that your future self will thank you for." You may be thinking, how many FAQs should I do? What if I think of a new one? What if someone asks me something and I haven't already written it? The answer to all of those is that it doesn't matter. Either explain the answer to the client or simply write it as your next FAQ. Don't think about the content you have available now, think about the content you will have available for your clients in six months' time. If you spent twenty minutes a day, five times a week writing 200 words on a FAQ, you would have a library of 24,000 words in six months. That's not bad for pre-written content. Rather than having to spend precious time on explaining this to people, you could just send them a PDF that compromises all the FAQs with a contents page so they can find things easily. How's that for customer service?

Getting your business to run on autopilot is the dream, but this dream takes a lot of hard work. Great things come from the accumulation of small habits over time. Those 200 words you write per day will eventually contribute to a book. You do have enough time in your day, and you can find the right words if you practice. There was probably a day where you weren't in the best of shape or that strong but look what lifting properly and applying consistency did for you. Writing becomes easier the more you do it. The people I hear say they're not good at writing don't seem to do much writing themselves. Find time in your day, be accountable to your goal, and let people read what you have to say. Just like people can't buy a package that doesn't exist, you also can't read an article or post that hasn't been written.

Planning and Structuring Studying

I had the mantra "The more you learn, the more you earn" for a long time. I thought that learning impressive but obscure facts contributed to being a better trainer and therefore earning more. However, if you can't apply what you've learned, it's not a great deal of use. When you set aside time to study, you need to research topics you will then be able to apply immediately in your next session. Think of it as a use it or lose it situation. You've just learned something, so it's fresh in your brain. Now you need to cement it by applying it in the field. Let's now look at the best times and best ways to study.

In 2015 I had a lady come to me asking to lose weight and do some knee rehabilitation. She'd had two ACL reconstructions (one in each knee) and needed some guidance on how to build back her strength and stability. When it comes to knee rehab, it's easy to think literally and presume training the knee joint is the best option. This may come in the form of leg extensions and step up variations. This isn't wrong, but if you dig out an anatomy book, you'll see that there are a lot of other muscles that also act on the knee and impact position. Therefore, you need to account for these muscles too. Knowing this is the case, you could then design exercises that strengthen or improve the length tension in these muscles, improving joint function as a by-product. A good trainer may know which exercises are good for the knee, like quad strengthening techniques. A great trainer knows which directions they need to set up the lines of pull in order to challenge a specific muscle in a specific range to identify a weakness or length tension issue. This all comes from learning anatomy but then seeing it in real life. My point is, you need to learn, apply, trial, and not be afraid to get things wrong. I'd be the first to admit that I've done exercises with people that haven't worked at all. I've even said to them there and then, "This isn't working optimally, let's try something else." It doesn't make you a bad person; everybody's human. Here is a list of my top tips on how to improve learning structure and recollection.

1.   Don't be a hero

Don't try to learn an entire textbook in a day. There are around 650 muscles in the human body. If you try to learn them all at once, you're not going to get very far. Learn one a day and you'll know them all in less than two years. Just learn one thing a day, that's it. Spend ten, twenty, or thirty minutes with a pad and pen writing notes and going over it several times.

2.   Make it easier to remember

If you Google the Latin language, you'll find that muscle anatomy is incredibly literal. For example, supra is above (Superman flying in the sky), infra is below (the one that isn't above), sub is underneath. The suffix "atus" mean "of the" or "belonging to". If we look at the scapula, we know it has a posterior spine that runs about a quarter of the way down parallel to the superior border.

Supraspinatus - above the spine
Infraspinatus - below the spine
Subscapularus - beneath the scapula

3.   Practice it, remember it, teach it

I teach a lot of my clients about muscles. I don't usually talk about the names of things or origins and insertion points, but I will say this muscle goes from here to here and it does this and this. It can be in complete layman's terms but that's all that matters. This is the best way to learn functional anatomy. Let's say you're looking at the infraspinatus. You know it causes external rotation of the humeral head (upper arm bone), which usually works synergistically with depression and medial adduction of the scapula. If you want to test someone's infraspinatus length tension, you would simply test their passive and active external rotation. If there is a restriction or discrepancy from one side to the other, you then know the position of the scapula won't be the same upon full external rotation (i.e. bottom of a pressing position). Therefore, you could conclude that pressing isn't the best exercise for this person to do, unless you have an intervention to change things there and then. What I love about anatomy is that it gives you the opportunity to problem solve and think critically. If you know where all the muscles are and what they do, your exercise set up, design, prescription, and cueing will all change.

4. See it everyday

People get impressed by the whole *Anatomy Trains* thing and the fascial lines. I know pretty much all of these by heart, which didn't actually come from studying, but from seeing. I have all the *Anatomy Trains* posters on my wall in my treatment room and so I see them every day whilst treating people. I know all the lines now purely from repeated exposure, not just sitting there with a pad and pen. Furthermore, it helps whilst treating people as I can trace along the lines and see how a restriction in one joint/muscle can lead to another. This combines the other component I spoke about: active learning and applying. For example, someone comes in with a hip issue that won't go away no matter how much other therapists have worked on it. After doing some assessments, you see they have poor strength in their tibialis anterior. This is impacting ankle mobility, which is affecting the gait and positioning of the ASIS. Therefore, if you work on the tibialis, you may relieve the pressure in the hip joint. Learn, apply, review, repeat.

5. Don't move topics

One of the most important things about learning is that you don't jump from one topic to the next. Yes, there are a lot of incredibly interesting subjects available to learn, but I must stress to only learn one field at once. If you try to master movement mechanics, the microbiome, and DNA transcription all at the same time, you're just going to be left frustrated. I know this all from first-hand experience. You've also got to think logically with this stuff. Talking about genetic coding sounds cool, but it really isn't going to achieve anything on the gym floor. When learning, think, "What will make me a better trainer?" After all, you're not a dietician, functional medicine specialist, or scientist, but a trainer. Funnily enough, it's all the stuff to do with training people. I don't think there's anything wrong with sporadic, specific learning. What I mean by this is when you have to study something in particular as a way of helping a client deal with an issue. You don't set out to learn it, you end up learning it by default because you really want to help people. If you asked a lot of the top coaches out there, they'd probably say the same. They acquired their wealth of knowledge through working with a plethora of different people with different issues. Learning how to overcome a problem there and then is invaluable. We often overlook the learn as you go aspect of coaching, but coaching itself is an art form that ultimately dictates the success of your business.

IN PERSON SKILLS

This section is designed to teach you what no traditional book can: experience. These are all the things I've learned purely from training people and not from a book or seminar. This isn't me saying, "You know it now, so you don't have to observe it yourself." Rather, pay attention to these things during your sessions, as they'll prove invaluable in the long run.

In-Person Skills: Listening

Keeping your mouth shut can make you money. As ridiculous as it sounds, knowing when and when not to speak can be the make or break behind building rapport with someone. If you want to get someone to like you, take you seriously, and do business with you, it pays to get good at listening. There is nothing more frustrating than having a conversation with someone who keeps interrupting you and isn't listening to a word you're saying. It's like they are only concerned about their agendas. I'm not going to start talking about neurotransmitters or brain science to explain this, I'm purely talking through experience. When people continue to cut me off when talking, I can't help but think how rude they are. You will always gravitate towards people who empathise with you. They are usually people who understand you. A person can't understand someone unless they listen to what you have to say. It's a step by step process. When someone only wants to speak and doesn't want to listen, they are clearly exhibiting that they are the main priority. This undervalues you and in turn, will annoy you. It doesn't matter how educated you are. It doesn't matter how good your results are. It doesn't matter how amazing your brand is or if you work in a world class facility, if people don't like you, they won't do business with you. When you meet a prospect client for the first time, it is your job—yes, job—to ask questions, listen patiently, and make notes. Pre-planned questions are always a good idea, but they can sometimes be counter-productive if unwarranted. Let's look at an example.

Trainer: "Have you had any injuries before?"

Potential client: "Yes, I was in a car crash two years ago and severely hurt my lower back. I was bed bound for two weeks and have hip pain whilst walking ever since."

Trainer nodding and taking notes: "And have you ever counted calories or used My Fitness Pal before?"

Think about this situation logically. This person has just told you a traumatic life event that impacts them on a daily basis. They will hold negative attachment to it and likely feel vulnerable or scared when mentioning it. When you don't even acknowledge what they're saying, it shows you haven't listened and that you don't really care. Having set questions is important but specifically responding to an answer with another provoking question will provide higher quality and more applicable information.

"How much does the pain affect you now?"
"Do you still think about the incident to this day?"

"Did you receive proper rehab support after the event?"
"What are your current stress levels like whilst dealing with the pain?"

These are a few follow up questions that move the conversation in an organic way. You'll find out more about the person and less facts or figures that don't correlate to much. Getting results with people is just psychology. They need to see that you care about them, that you can help them, and that you're listening to them. Any good coach knows that you must react, not predict. When looking to get lean, you can't just take out 100 calories a week until you're shredded. You must see how the body's responding, monitor certain markers, and then react based on what the current situation is showing. This is coaching. It makes things truly individual. If you just follow set protocols, you are not catering for a person's needs. It's rare that you'll win someone over in a conversation or consultation through flaunting your knowledge. If they say something that is met with a line from a textbook or research paper, they'll usually feel confused or intimidated. If what they say is met with a question wanting to know more about their situation, or perhaps a solution to a common problem they're having, you're much more likely to build rapport and gain their trust. These rules are universal. I believe that listening is one of the most important parts of a relationship. When you ask your partner how their day was, listen to what they have to say. Ask them a follow up question. It shows you're listening and it shows you care.

Before looking into advance sales techniques, the psychology of selling or other money-making tools, ensure you are doing the basics right. You shoulder never interrupt someone during a consultation when first speaking to them, especially if they're talking about something important. Learn to listen. It will make you money.

This section will cover concepts you may not have thought about before. It's so you can fully grasp what your clients go through and the reasons they may not be progressing the way you'd want them to. In my opinion, 90% of the time, it's not the training or methodology, it's the lifestyle demands that carry a higher priority that get in the way.

First let's look at body transformations. I used to be a real hater on body transformations. "Yeah but they're unsafe, that person won't be healthy, they probably took a load of drugs and didn't eat much" and so on. Truth is, I was just jealous because I'd never achieved one of these transformations before and I'd never gotten seriously lean myself. It was all a mystery to me. The fact of the matter is, you can be as smart as you like, but the people who get the most leads in this industry will be the ones producing the most before and after pictures. That's just the way it is.

I've never wanted to be a body transformation coach. Strength and biomechanics have always been more interesting and fun for me. This being said, the majority of people I deal with do want to lose body fat and look better. Therefore, if I don't know how to do this, I'm missing out on business, which isn't smart. Before I talk to you about your clients, I want you to fully understand what one of these incredible transformations takes. My biggest downfall as a coach has always been being too nice—not dropping food enough, not prescribing cardio, not pushing them out of their comfort zone. I will tell you here and now that you WILL have to do all those things to get people to look visually different. Unfortunately, with some general population clients, they can lose 2–3 stone and not look any different in a picture. They may move better, sleep better, and feel better, but because of a lack of muscle mass, they don't end up looking too different from their initial shot. You could devise the best write up in the world and talk about health markers, etc., but it may not suffice for the fickle viewers of the internet. When you want to produce a jaw dropping general population transformation, this person will need to reach "The Darkness" as my business partner Jay and I call it. This is when calories are low, output is high, irritability is rife, and things just aren't that pleasant. It's not nice and it's not particularly healthy. I must add though, achieving low levels of body fat whilst maintaining good health takes years. You can either drop a lot of body fat quickly and sacrifice health, or you can do it safely and sacrifice time. Unless you are a multi-millionaire with surplus amounts of time and funds, it's difficult to drop an insane amount of fat quickly and retain perfect health. You have to take them to a whole new level of discomfort and you must explain that to them initially. Never lie to them about the hard work it will take.

When I first started as a coach and was living at my parents' house, I used to get frustrated at how my clients weren't progressing. I couldn't get my head around why they weren't losing weight or sticking to the plan. Since my situation has changed, I fully understand how it can be incredibly difficult to prioritise health, diet, and childcare at the same time. I think it's both naive and disrespectful for young singletons on social media to say to people, "You are fat because fitness isn't a priority." When you're a parent, your sole purpose in life should be the happiness and wellbeing of your children. It's the most selfless thing you can do to ensure they have a nice childhood. When trainers say, "You watch an hour of TV a night when you could be training," they don't appreciate that the parent may have been up since 4:30am, done a full day's work, got home, made tea, bathed, and put the kids to bed and then have one hour alone with their spouse to chill out.

The reality is that life *is* difficult for people based on their work and home environment. If you don't understand this, you don't understand your client and you'll never fully understand how to cater for them. If you can't cater for them, you'll lose their business. It's like if I were watching people run a marathon but have never ran more than a mile in my life. If someone was struggling the last five miles and I shouted, "Why don't you run a bit faster?" I'd look like a bit of an idiot. This is, however, what you are doing when you say, "Why haven't you stuck to your macros?" to a parent who has three kids and a full time job. You try throwing away two chicken nuggets and a bit of ketchup whilst on 1,700 calories a day! In April 2019 I decided to undertake photoshoot prep so I could fully understand what it was like to be both a full-time parent and "enter the darkness" at the same time. It's not nice. In fact, it can be horrible at times. If I were to impart this on any person, I would first make sure they know what they're getting themselves into and second, know that I'm going to have to be on hand to coach them as best as I possibly can. The biggest issue with the fitness industry isn't the diet and training methodology. It's not the crossfit or the keto or the 5:2 intermittent fasting intravenous coconut oil diet; it's the fact that you have a plethora of trainers who don't understand the people they're trying to communicate to. It's like you're speaking Spanish to a room full of Chinese people. One or two may understand, but the majority are going to look at you and think, "What the hell are they going on about?" Think about how you can communicate to your audience. You might communicate differently if your client wants a transformation, not weight loss, and by that I mean rippling abs and sub-10% body fat, then you will need to explain to them what they're going to have to put themselves through. If you haven't done it or don't understand it yourself, maybe you're not the best person for them to be working with. Understand your client. Appreciate what they go through. Never lie to them about what's required to achieve a goal.

In-Person Skills: Understanding the process

Should PTs be ripped? Should we walk around the gym at 5% body fat all year round, six-packs out, pecs (or glutes if you are female) flaunted like peacocks during mating season? The answer is no, just no. Being ripped doesn't make you a good coach and from my experience, the coaches who have an easier time of naturally staying lean struggle to properly connect with their general population clients. They can't seem to understand their problems. This being said, getting lean at some point of your career is useful.

I'm not saying you should be shredded by any means, but if you don't ever go through some sort of rigorous diet prep at some stage of your career, you're missing out on one of the most valuable lessons in understanding your clients. I believe that the body works in set points. It finds homeostasis and protects it for everything it's worth. Your body doesn't like change; it means it has to adapt, and adaptation can be pretty difficult. Once you've been lean or muscular for a certain amount of time, it takes more effort to fall out of your habits than it does to keep them. Our brains work in a "rinse and repeat" manner. The more you do something, the easier it becomes to do. Now when someone is overweight and out of shape, their brain will believe that the easiest option for them is to continue being overweight and out of shape. Change won't come naturally and they will encounter some form of resistance (in many people's case, a lot of resistance). People like this need guidance and this is why good PTs are worth their weight in gold. You are not an accessory or nicety for the affluent. You are contributing positively to society by keeping people healthy. The way I see it, the will power, changes in habits, and lifestyle alterations that take your average joe from 30% body fat to 15% are similar to what takes your average PT from 12% body fat down to 5%. You need to make some substantial lifestyle changes and be consistent with them.

Let's now talk about you, the trainer. You will probably find it easy to get up in the morning. You probably train 3–5 times a week with good intensity. You probably hit your protein target, 2 litres of water, and 10,000 steps a day with ease. It is like a default setting for you. You probably also like the odd indulgence at the weekend. You'll have a glass of wine with your spouse, the odd pizza, maybe a family meal where you were liberal with your dessert choices. It's cool; I'll be the first to tell you that I do this too. My point being, most PTs are

80/20. We do all the things we need to do right but are lenient at the right times. This is how you should be.

However, when you're looking to get lean, and I mean really lean, this all goes out the window. If you have a photo shoot or competition coming up, the wine, dark chocolate, and balance goes out the window. You must stick to the plan, otherwise you're not going to look how you'd like. The camera doesn't lie during a photo shoot, trust me. This is where the roles reverse. All the little indulgences must go. If they don't, your physique will show it. You have to make some significant lifestyle changes that push you out of your comfort zone. This is similar to, you guessed it, your general population clients when they first start off with you. Some will come to you only eating 40–50g of protein a day and eating 100–120g will seem like a mission impossible. Some will only drink teas or coffees and tell you they don't like water. Some will have a diet that is 90% carbohydrates. Some will do less than 1,000 steps per day. Some will not have done any form of exercise in twenty years. I could go on. Even though the stuff that you do seems natural, the things you want your clients to do are humungous changes in their daily regime. Some are in fact unfathomable for certain clients.

"Meat for breakfast? Meat? For breakfast? Are you insane?"

This is why it's essential that at some point of your career you understand what they have to go through in those initial phases. I'm not saying you should get ripped because PTs need to be ripped (we don't), but the process of getting extremely lean will provide you with an incredible insight into what your clients will go through. Whilst dieting, I've gone to bed hungry. I've been cranky, my energy has suffered, and I've felt physically and mentally tired for weeks. I've daydreamed about food yet found my appetite decreasing. I've obsessed about my weight and got scared when it's not changed. I've meticulously stuck to my calories and done 15,000 steps a day on weekends. Being truthful, it wasn't very nice. I didn't enjoy it. This is exactly how some of your clients will feel when first implementing the basics of nutrition such as calorie control, protein intake, and energy expenditure. The purpose of this section isn't to explain to you what it's like to get lean. I'm telling you that to truly understand the process, you must take yourself through it yourself.

Imagine this scenario. A woman comes to me for PT when she's six-months pregnant. I train her for two months but towards the end of her pregnancy she starts to get anxiety about giving birth for the first time. I constantly reassure her saying she'll be fine and it doesn't hurt that much and that it'll be over before she knows it. Do you think she'll really take what I have to say on board? Not a chance! Why? Because I've never given birth. You can't truly guide someone on a journey you've never been on before. It's like the blind leading the blind. You need to understand their worries, their challenges, and the best ways to psychologically and physically overcome obstacles.

To summarise, being ripped does not make you a good trainer. However, going from great shape to insane shape takes a lot of sacrifice. These sacrifices are similar to that of what your general population clients must do in the initial phases of their diet plan to see significant changes. If you want to truly understand what they're going through, therefore making you a more skilled coach, you must take yourself through a similar experience with similar sacrifices and emotions. One of the biggest separations that impairs the ability to relate with your client is that you are already in shape. People bond over similar experiences. If you know what someone is going through or are going through the same experience simultaneously, you'll build a tremendous amount of rapport with them, which will increase the likelihood of them achieving results.

In-Person Skills: Coming out of your shell

Personal training; it contains two words, both of which give you a good indication of what you need to be good at. Yes, training knowledge is important, but it's only half as important as knowing how to interact with people on a personal level. If you don't learn how to do this, you're leaving business growth on the table. If you want to get better as a coach, I believe it's best to throw yourself in the deep end and work with the general public as much as possible in any setting. During the initial draft of this book on my Facebook page, one member asked whether they should take group exercise classes. They were new to the industry and not sure whether it was a good or bad idea. Now let me begin by saying that it is possible to open a can of worms with group classes. They are, in some cases, a crime against proper training form and may make you cringe based on some people's technique.

I remember my first circuit class in a commercial gym. It was rife with ridiculously shallow squats, flared elbow press ups, and neck straining crunches galore. It was scary. A lot of these people were probably doing more damage than good. Putting shocking training form aside, there is a reason you must do some form of group exercise class at least once in your coaching career. It's simply character building. The internet is a dangerous place and due to generational issues, it's possible to call yourself an expert without actually interacting with people. Knowledge makes you knowledgeable. An expert is someone with excellent knowledge who's helped hundreds, if not thousands, of people. You can only do this by putting yourself out there.

There will be some of you reading this now who are intent on being the best trainer you can be. You want to be "perfect" to a degree and want to learn as much as possible so you can get the best results possible. I'm going to tell you now to stop worrying. There is no such thing as the perfect trainer. Anyone who claims to be is giving a false pretence. I still make mistakes and am far from the completed article. I'm just a bit better at what I do than I used to be. My point is, you need to fail to get better and group classes provide the perfect opportunity for this. Let me explain with another little hypothetical analogy.

Rupert has just come out of university. He received a first in sports & exercise science and is now doing a master's in physiology part time. He eats a perfectly clean diet, trains impeccably well, lives and breathes bodybuilding, and studies biochemistry and anatomy for at least an hour a day. His dream is to be one of the best coaches in the world and he has just started working a commercial gym facility. Ryan is an ex-footballer who had to give up his playing career due to a knee injury. He rehabbed it through weight training and thought he'd learn to be a PT as he got bitten by the gym bug when doing all those leg extensions. He's not very academic, slightly dyslexic, and very much a jack the lad who still likes to go out on weekends. He has just started in the same gym as Rupert and they are both trying to build a client base.

Rupert patrols the gym floor looking to correct people who aren't training properly. He plucks up the courage to offer assistance to those training "sub optimally" and explains the importance of moment arms, lines of pull, and movement profiles during an exercise. These people are really impressed with his knowledge and say, "Wow, I can really feel that working now. Thank you." However, after a month, Rupert still hasn't had any sign ups.

Ryan isn't exactly a book worm; he gets asked to cover a group class circuit one day so decides to go for it. His witty banter makes him a hit with the ladies and the men love the fact he's an ex-footballer who can talk about beer and sport. He wings his group class putting on an old circuit session he remembers back in the day, training the hell out of everyone. They all leave absolutely knackered but with a smile on their faces. Ryan has four new clients by the end of the month.

Group exercise classes are the best way to show off your personality. This is a huge aspect of your business. People will buy from you if they trust and like you. If they don't get the chance to get to know you properly, how will they figure this out? Don't be scared if people in your classes aren't doing the most perfectly executed biomechanically aligned squat. This doesn't make you a bad coach and defeats the whole point of group exercise. The people are there for the atmosphere and fun you can create, not necessarily the workout you can provide. Yes, doing things safely is vital, but the energy you can provide in a room is even more important. If you were doing a class and saw a woman doing an exercise poorly, go up and give her some cues on how she can improve her technique. If she continues to do things poorly then she will require PT to go over these things in more detail. It is your job to let her know you provide those skills and it's her job to figure out you're the person to see—that's it. I've taught spin classes, circuit classes, aqua aerobics, exercise the music classes, you name it. I've absolutely smashed some of these classes and some have gone down like a fart in a lift. Honestly, some of the classes I've done have been an absolute disaster, but that's the point; it's character building. You can either take it on the chin, brush yourself off, and do another, or you can sit behind a laptop, study all day, and call yourself an online expert. If you want to get busy in a one-to-one setting, learn how to deal with people face to face. I'm telling you now that I categorically wouldn't be the trainer I am today without the massive fails I've gone through in the past. And believe me, there have been a lot.

If you can do a class whilst on shift and get paid for it, do it. Think of it as a way of getting paid for exposure. Learn people's names, try to make them laugh, ask them about their training and their lives, and generally take an interest in them. All these things make you a better coach and will prove invaluable one day. Knowledge is knowing a heavy quarter squat may put undesirable shearing forces on a forty-year-old guy's knees whilst he's training. Wisdom is knowing that telling him what he's doing is wrong will only lead to "Pipe down, son, I've been training since you were in nappies." You have to learn how to deal with people and group training is an excellent opportunity for this. You'll get just as much from stepping out of your comfort zone and in front of a room of people as you would from burying your nose in a book all day. Don't be afraid to fail. The best failures lead to the biggest growth.

In-Person Skills: Perfection is not achievable

People always like it when they can associate with someone. Having a level of rapport immediately creates a sense of connection, which builds trust. I want to assure you all that despite me constantly pursuing being the best coach possible, it's not actually something that you can do.

I have a client whose goal is hypertrophy. I get him to do a core potentiation warm up, get him to do some feeder sets, and then train him as hard as I can. Given he's trained with me for six years, I can push him pretty close to failure on a lot of exercises. Despite me doing everything you'd expect a good PT to do—being prompt, having his programme ready for him, timing his rest intervals, instructing every rep—this still didn't stop my client from spending three minutes of a rest period telling me all about the latest reality dating show. He got so engrossed in telling me the latest gossip that we ended up going over his rest period and taking a three minute break instead of ninety seconds. I was still timing the rest interval, I just couldn't stop him from talking. Another client I had owns multiple businesses. He's extremely busy and I can see why. He has a law firm, real estate, an insurance firm, and five kids. You can imagine how switched on he is all the time. Whilst I was training him, he had to take a phone call four times. He took the calls during rest periods, so it wasn't rude, and always apologised by saying, "I need to take this," which I understood. I'd been working with him for two years and know first-hand how busy he is.

So, does talking about dating shows and letting a client take a phone call make me a bad PT? I'll let you be the judge. All I will say is that you've got to remember that you're working with people, not robots, and that having a personal element to things is incredibly important. The fact of the matter is, a lot of people will train with you for years because they like you, not just because you're a good trainer. This does not in mean you can slack, get lazy, or be unprofessional; it just means you shouldn't beat yourself up if you're not perfect in your own self-critical eye. As long as your foundations are right, give yourself a bit of leeway.

What are the foundations if you're wondering?

- Always be on time
- Always be dressed and smell well
- Always have a stopwatch
- Never go on your phone during a session
- Always have the session planned
- Don't let them complete one single rep without your tuition or guidance.

If you do those, don't worry if you stray off the topic and even make your client laugh every now and again. I've been extremely fortunate to work with PTs who've been training people for 10–20 years. What you gain in these years isn't just training knowledge, it's the skill of how to work with people. Nothing can teach you this, and some things come with age. You have to appreciate that coaching is about accommodating for their personality and providing them with the support they need, not just training.

If you ever doubt yourself due to seeing a "How to Spot a Bad PT" post online, take solace in the fact that the person posting is just making a detrimental move for their own business. Knocking people down to elevate your own status is never wise. It's not integral and it shows that you're focused (or even worried) about your competition. I fully understand that there probably are some sub-par trainers out there, but there's nothing I can do about that. They don't give personal trainers a bad name, you give yourself a bad name. As long as you put out the best content and portray yourself in the best way possible, you don't have to worry about anyone else.

Audi is a great brand of car. I would say they're on the closer side of high end and build everything from family to supercars. However, what would your feelings towards Audi be like if you saw a billboard saying, "BMWs are overpriced and unreliable, buy an Audi"? Aggressive, unneeded, petty, immature? Remember, content creation is your opportunity to bring either positivity or negativity into the world. Say something positive, receive positive back. Say something negative, guess what happens? If someone has the time to do a video or post on how bad other people are, it just shows that they have nothing better to do with their time than berate other people. If they were smart (or busy) they'd spend this time training people, writing programmes, or creating useful content for their target audience.

The perfect PT doesn't exist, so don't worry if you ever have self-doubt about yourself because a client wants to talk about their favourite TV show or an argument with a spouse when they should be training. It's just part of life. Stick to the foundations of what you should be doing but adapt your sessions around what the person requires the most. Some people may talk your ear off, some people may not talk at all. Your goal is to ensure that regardless of how much talking is done, they still complete the set workout to the right intensity. You may at times have to tell people to stop talking and focus, but this is a people skill you will develop with time and practise. You should have every intention of being as best as you can be but know that being the perfect trainer isn't always realistic.

In-Person Skills: Learn just as much from them as they learn from you

Would you say you're the average of the people you spend the most time with? I would. You pick up mannerisms, ways of thinking, likes, dislikes, and habits from those around you. It makes sense if you think about it. You become the product of what you're exposed to most frequently. If you bear this in mind, how much of an effect do you think your clients have on your personality, mindset, and approach to running your business?

I have people who see me 3–5 times per week. Let's say on average this is four hours. We will also chat via the phone to go over anything they may need help with, meaning interaction time will be quite high. The fact of the matter is, I see some of my clients way more than I see my friends and family. I believe that it's human nature to find companionship in any form.

You'll warm to those you spend time with and eventually build relationships. Your clients will inevitably mould you and change your traits. It's an unavoidable process that highlights why you should choose who you work with carefully. I'm not saying you should turn people away, but if you get bad vibes from someone and they ask for some sort of deal, it is essential that you don't work with them. No amount of money is worth someone poisoning your mindset.

What does this make me? Well, I'm a commercial property lawyer, property developer, law firm owner, and stock exchange investor—at least in theory. I earn anything from between £100,000 to a million pounds per year. I have over seventy years' experience in the real world, and I'm well educated, wise, and know the mistakes of rash or miscalculated views.

What's my point? You have the skills to train people; they have the skills to educate you on anything else. A lot of the extremely useful information I've used to grow my business has come directly from my clients. I know I've spoken frequently about the importance of being professional, timing rest intervals, and training people properly; however, I recommend never to miss out on an opportunity to learn from your clients. The incredible thing about personal training is that some of these people would charge several hundreds of pounds for an hour of their time, yet here they are, talking to you, telling you everything they know, and you're getting paid. I'm not saying you should ask clients, "What's the most valuable information you have to offer?" However, when someone speaks, listen. People like to talk, and they love to talk about things they are good at. If people are seeing you multiple times per week, they'll more than likely be pretty decent at making money.

For many people, the growth of their business comes at the expense of their health. When they start to work with you and see improvements in their body composition, energy levels, and fitness, they will be extremely indebted. I've had some clients who've turned around and said, "You don't understand how much you've helped me." That really affects me. I thought

I was following standard protocol—talking about calories, stress management, and sleep—but this isn't known information for a lot of people. If there's a case where a client wants to repay you, I wouldn't go for the option of using their holiday home or going to an executive sports game with them. Instead, learn from them. Go for a coffee and ask all about how they got to where they are today, what are the most valuable things they learned, and what would they advise to their younger self.

When my law firm manager client lost his first stone, he repaid me by giving me an hour with his IT team learning all about search engine optimisation (SEO). We went through how to maximise a website for it to increase the rankings on Google organically. That was extremely useful for me considering I went on to write around fifty articles on my website that year. One of my other clients, who I've trained for seven years, used to take me out for a coffee and we'd chat all about the fitness industry and what he liked and disliked. This was great as I got a first-hand insight in to what people outside of fitness think about influencers on social media. This was invaluable. He'd say, "I like this guy and that guy," to which I'd reply, "Yeah, but that's really basic information." His response was, "Yeah, I know. That's why I like it." It showed me what general punters will think of the content I put out and why it'll go over their head a lot of the time. This client also told me one thing that stayed with me to this day: *"You get in a lift with someone. You have the time it takes in the lift to sell your services. What do you say?"*

Erm…

I remember when he first asked me this and it caught me a little off guard. I immediately wanted to go into greater detail and try to over complicate things to sound more advanced. This isn't wise when you only have a short space of time. He then went on to explain that on social media, you have around seven seconds to get someone's attention. After that, they'll scroll on to the next more entertaining video of a cat playing the piano. Time is precious, so make sure you know how to communicate your services. This brief excerpt from a conversation re-shaped the way I thought about social media and my marketing strategies. It can take just one person to completely revolutionise your thinking. I would definitely attribute a lot of my development to working with business-minded individuals. If I'd just seen these people as numbers or before and after pictures, I would have missed out on some valuable information that allowed me to grow. It's incredibly important to train people hard and be strict during sessions, but it's critical to develop the skill of knowing when to let people speak. Even if it's not direct financially driven advice, the wisdom these people can give you may change your outlook on a lot of areas, be it how to become more business minded or when to recognise you're going to burn yourself out from working too many hours and not enough sleep.

HOW TO KNOW WHEN YOU'RE
WORKING TOO MUCH

What's the point of working hard? No, I'm actually asking you. Why should we get up early, study, train, eat well, and be diligent with our time? What does it achieve? I bet you've never been asked that before. I'm here to tell you now that I'll have been ten times more guilty of working for the sake of working than you ever will. Again, like many agendas in this book, I just want to make sure that you don't make the same mistakes as I did.

Finding out people's 'why' usually lies within their past. For me, it boils down to one specific moment. It was ten years ago, during my first visit to university studying sport and exercise science. I say "studying" but I did very little of that. Believe it or not, I wasn't the best student the first-time around at university. I got a job as a bar man and spent most of my time in the gym. I used to work until 6:00am and it played havoc with my body clock. I remember my parents coming to visit me one Sunday and me being physically unable to stay awake at the table when we went out for food. I think my head dipped into my Sunday lunch a few times. The turning point came one afternoon. It was 2:00pm and I was lay in bed starring at the ceiling. I was so tired that I didn't even have the energy to get up and walk to the kitchen. I had to drop out of uni due to my grades and living away from home had got the best of me. I had no routine, was exhausted all the time, and had no path or career prospects. I hated that feeling. I felt like I had no purpose and I needed to do something. By divine intervention (a random email that popped up in my spam), I decided to apply to do a personal training qualification that summer and ended up jumping straight into the deep end. I had always wanted to be a personal trainer. I even wrote it on my career form in school when I was 17. I just thought you had to first do three years at uni before applying. Turns out that wasn't the case.

Fast forward four years and I went self-employed at as a PT for the first time. It wasn't as safe as working in a commercial gym and I quickly realised that if you're not productive with lead generation and developing content, your income is going to suffer. I started to write more, work early, work late, train harder, and build my brand to grow my business. My income improved, but it wasn't calculated. I wasn't paying attention to how I was growing; I just knew I was heading the right direction. I correlated effort to earnings, which was both a good and bad mindset. I knew if I worked hard, I earned more. I now have the luxury of knowing this isn't actually the case. I was just addressing an emotion, not earning more money. I increased my earning *in spite* of what I was doing, not because of it. I never again wanted to have that feeling of worthlessness I felt whilst staring at my dorm room ceiling. I masked that feeling by keeping myself busy with tasks and being in perpetual go mode. The problem was, as this mindset was growing, so was the internet. Along came faster internet connections, smart phone apps, podcasts, and Instagram. As funny as it sounds, these were just concepts when I first qualified as a PT. The birth of the cyber world meant people were hungrier for content and I was determined to feed them.

Now I'd estimate that I've easily uploaded half a million words online over the years. I started content production in 2011 and know that in 2017 alone I uploaded 125,000 words (I counted that one). By law of averages and given the amount of time I dedicate to writing, half a million will have been surpassed quite comfortably. The thing is, I never monetised or at least capitalised on growing a market. I was extremely busy keeping up with this enormous quota I'd set myself, but it wasn't achieving much. When it boiled down to it, for a large majority of that time, one-to-one PT was the only thing that made me money. I was just working for working's sake.

That all may sound a little contraindicative based on previous sections: "But Chris, I thought you want us to develop our brand and create content!" I do, I couldn't recommend it enough. However, it needs to be done efficiently, accurately, and not at the expense of your health. Your work ethic shouldn't scare people; your results and content production should. I'd be more impressed by the person who works up until 3:00pm each day yet releases multiple articles, podcasts, and results, than the person who gets up at 4:30am and goes to bed at 11:00pm but has half as much to show for it. You know when you're working too much when your ability to produce content or deliver a session reduces. When sleep is impaired, cognition is poor, and you rely on stimulants to get through the day, you know it's time to reassess things. Just like a strength athlete needs a de-load once performance drops, you need a break from work when performance starts to suffer. No one wants to train with a tired PT full of excuses. People pay more for excellence, so it's in your best interest to be excellent.

I've now found that the more you work, the less you get done. If you give yourself too much time to do a task, productivity drops. I call it "deadline syndrome". We all know that deadline feeling we got at school or uni. We have a 10,000-word project due in two weeks that we haven't even started. One week, to three days, to one day out, we work ourselves stupid and eventually complete the work in a caffeinated, frantic state. We get work done because there is a time constraint and urgency. If we extrapolate one of these factors and utilise it, your productivity but most of all lifestyle will improve.

Once you've established that your work quality or content production is dropping, you then need to create deadlines for when you're allowed to work. If you're allowed to work at any point of the day, the urgency to get a task done reduces. If you have the mindset that you'll work on this task until the early hours of the morning until it gets done, there is an unregulated time allowance. This decreases productivity. If you change this to working on it until 7:00pm then turning your phone and laptop off, your work efficiency will improve dramatically. You've created urgency and we work better under pressure. It's important that you create a work curfew.

We as trainers can be messy with our time. Working in the gym until 9:00pm and then typing out client diets and programmes until midnight is going to negatively impact your health and nothing more. You will have had time in your day to complete those tasks, you just didn't apply enough urgency in that situation to get it done. You either got distracted on your phone or chatting to friends. I'm not saying you can't do these things; I'm just saying they have to take a back seat to your most important priorities. To put it simply, if you work past 8:00pm, you're working hard but you're not working smart. Longevity and avoiding burning out favours the latter. The magic happens once you learn how to work both smart and hard.

If you're reading this and thinking, I *am* actually that busy with one-to-one clients that I don't have time in the day, then fair enough. I admire your work ethic, but I think you're missing out on business opportunities. If you're doing 10–12 sessions a day, 5–6 days a week, you should have put your prices up a long time ago. Volume indicates affordability and not is not ideal when you're a person who trades time for money. You always need to evaluate how you can increase your profit per unit sold. If you don't, you'll become stuck working the same long hours for the same money. The main take away from this section is that you need to have delegated times to work on one task. This is explained well in the Gary Keller book *The One Thing*. When sitting down for a gap in your day, you must have one objective to complete and nothing more. Do not cross contaminate and go from one area to another. It shouldn't be one client programme, one social media post, fifteen minutes studying. It should be to complete all your programmes in one sitting. You have ninety minutes to do so, with phone breaks only allowed for five-minute intervals every 25–30 minutes. If you don't complete the tasks, you then have until your next delegated break either later that day or the next day. If you don't get your work done, you have to have the awkward conversation with your client about not getting their programme to them because you didn't have time. This should be motivation enough to ensure you don't lose track of time and get distracted. Once you get the hang of this, you'll realise how much your late nights and feeling of being overwhelmed were unneeded. You're capable of completing a lot more work than you think, a lot quicker than you think. You just haven't created enough urgency to do so. Don't get addicted to the feeling of needing to work like I did. Get addicted to the feeling of getting stuff done.

As you are now familiar with the concept of income delegation, you'll be aware that once your wage, rent, and tax have been accounted for, there's not a great deal left over. The amount of money this equates to will depend on your total income, so the more you earn the more this amount would be. If you have 2.5-5% aside, I would create something called a reset fund. This is where you save money to do something on an 8–12-week basis where you completely spoil yourself. It may sound self-indulgent, but mini breaks and relaxation are incredibly important to your development. If you neglect them, your work will suffer. If your work suffers, your income suffers. Therefore, you can see their importance.

If I asked you when muscles grow, most people would say it's when they recover. It's the gym work that stimulates development but the recovery time and nutrition that leads to growth. It's the same with business. You can't see how well your business is doing until you remove yourself from it for a brief period. If you're constantly immersed in it, all you can see is the wheels spinning and the chaos of everyday life. It's not until you can take a step back that you see what really needs work. I would recommend that every eight weeks, you (and your partner if you have one) book in for some quality time at a spa day or stay overnight in a hotel. Don't take your phone, don't take your laptop. Completely detach from the outside world. If you take anything, make it a pad of paper. Write down your thoughts, how happy you are with your progress, and where you want to take your business. Relax, unwind, and gain clarity. Just like we respond better to daily time constraints, it's powerful to have breaks in your calendar and things to look forward to—whether it's one meal out with your spouse a month, a spa day every eight weeks, or two holidays a year. There is so much more to life than working and it's incredibly important you see this. Ironically, your greatest epiphanies in how you can maximise your business will come once you detach yourself from it.

The purpose of this book is to help you create a business that complements your lifestyle, not hinders it. That's one of the biggest principles of the 5 x 5 rule. Twenty-five personal training sessions a week, five hours on educational development, and five hours on brand development. Keep it precise and to the point. You don't work more than this, but you don't work less either. You develop your business within the hours you set and then live a relaxed, fulfilled life in the time in between.

BRAND DEVELOPMENT

THE PURPOSE OF BUILDING A FOLLOWING

Nowadays if you're a personal trainer, you're also a brand—or at least, you have the ability to make yourself a brand. With social media, YouTube, and personal training assistance data bases, you can create your own company with an identity, ethos, and mission. It's exciting, but it can be daunting. Where do you begin? In this section, I'll be talking you through all the elements that have helped me build my brand.

Before I begin, I'd like to talk to you about "The Dwayne Johnson shout out" theory of brand development. Don't worry if you're unfamiliar with this term, it's something I made up. It will shed some light on the importance of brand development but also cross reference back to prioritising the right parts of your business. Consider this hypothetical situation. It's 9:00pm, you've had a busy day, and just finished your last client. You get home, shower, get in bed, and check your phone for the last time. At 7:00pm, in between clients, you uploaded a meme likening peak time at the gym to the 2000 Royal Rumble and shared it on your Instagram page. It's gotten a few likes and interactions, but nothing major. You think nothing of it, turn off your phone, and go to sleep. The next morning you wake up, brush your teeth, turn on your phone, and do the usual What's App and social media checks. You go on Instagram and notice you have half a million new followers. You jolt in disbelief. At first, you assume it's merely a glitch and that it will correct itself shortly. You close down the app and go on it again. To your bemusement, it's still there. Your following has increased by 500,000 in less than eight hours. So what happened?

You sift through your inbox and see that Dwayne "The Rock" Johnson saw the meme you shared and put it in his story. It was followed by a clip of him saying, "Shout out to (your name) for reminding me of this wrestling victory. That was a great day, thank you brother." You tagged him in the post but never thought anything of it. However, due to this interaction, your Instagram account has now just been seen by over 125 million people. How amazing would that be? But here's the thing I want you to think about. Although it may look amazing to have this new-found mini fame, does it actually mean anything? How long will these new followers stick around? After a week, would you drop down to 400,000, then 300,000? Would you be able to maintain their attention and provide them with value? Enter brand development. The first stage of building a personal training business is getting busy as a one-to-one coach and developing a reputation locally. The evolution of a personal training business is to monetise your expertise by creating a passive income stream or a product that can be utilised by a high number of people. If you do neither of these, having a lot of followers is irrelevant. If someone were to randomly land on your page, you need to think, "What can they consume?" Is it articles, videos, podcasts, or programmes? How do you create fans? This is essentially what brand development is: becoming known for having a certain message or product.

In Daniel Priestley's 2015 book *Oversubscribed*, he talks about the importance of reaching people on multiple levels. This is over an array of different mediums that boost legitimacy. I remember reading this back in 2016, which really prompted my devotion to setting up a podcast. In 2017, I made sure I wrote 100,000 words of content on my website that year. In 2018, I set up an online training company, and in 2019 I released my first passive income product in the form of this book. If each time I now gain a follower, they can read my articles, listen to my podcasts, work with me via online training, or purchase reading material. Having an audience now serves a purpose. Brand development isn't just about making money. It will contribute to your ability to earn money, but the way I see it, it's the impression you leave on the world. Your persona, your style, and your message is like a contribution to society. It therefore bares a tremendous amount of value if it has a positive impact on someone's wellbeing. There's nothing more exciting than knowing you have the ability to bring value to people's lives.

SETTING UP YOUR OWN PODCAST

Podcasts are quickly becoming one of the most popular and accessible formats of content consumption around. They provide an easy way for your audience to get used to your voice, message, and personality. In essence, you're allowing people to get to know you without ever meeting them. Here's everything I've learned from setting up my own show and building an audience.

Back in 2016, I was very into The Joe Rogan Podcast. As one of the world's biggest shows, it attracted the smartest people in the fitness industry. I remember getting excited when it was announced that certain people would be on the show. I thought, "Wouldn't it be cool to do something like this myself?" Almost three years on and I've surpassed a hundred episodes. I've been fortunate to have some great guests on the show and have educated myself immensely by chatting with some great minds. Podcasts add layers to your business. If you'd like to set up your own podcast, here are my top tips for you.

1. Put your doubts to one side

"Why would anyone want to listen to me?" Don't worry, I had the exact same thought. Many people, including myself, may feel they have imposter syndrome by setting up a podcast. They may feel it's a bit self-righteous, as if you have all the answers and like to think you know what you're talking about. You may feel you're a nobody in a world breamed with intellect and talent. I'm here to tell you this isn't the case. People can't buy from you if you don't have a product. People can't listen to you if you don't have a show. If you don't shoot, you don't score. There is absolutely nothing stopping your show from being a phenomenon; it all depends on whether you start it or not. The people making waves in this industry are not necessarily the smartest. They are the ones most confident in their ability to address a room. If you speak with authority and cast your doubts to one side, you have just as much right as the next person to start a show.

2. Techie bits: Hosting and recording

A hosting website is where you upload your podcasts. It means they can easily get on to iTunes and Spotify. I've found Buzzsprout to be the best hosting site and a lot easier to use. If the figures are accurate, I'm currently averaging a thousand listens per episode, which I'm pretty happy with. It will also show you where people are listening geographically. Due to the guests I've had on, quite a few of my listeners are based in America and Australia, which is pretty cool.

When speaking to guests, I prefer Zoom to Skype. Although Skype is free, I've found that the sound quality and connection isn't the best, whereas Zoom tends to be consistent. Using both Buzzsprout and Zoom does have a fee of £17.99 and £14.39 a month. This means your podcast out-goings will be about £33 a month.

I use Quicktime player audio when recording a podcast. I simply press record and then press finish recording when we're done. It's that simple. Make sure you have the volume all the way down, as otherwise it'll record a reverb and you'll hear echoing noise when you listen to it back. Once you've recorded your podcast, I recommend uploading the raw taping to Dropbox immediately after you've finished the conversation. It is then safe in cyber space and can be downloaded if anything happens to your laptop or hard drive. I once did a podcast with a world-renowned doctor and managed to delete it whilst clearing some data off my laptop. I spent about £40 on software to recover the data but had no luck. Fortunately, he was amazing about it and agreed to come back on the show to re-record. I record my intros and outros separately on a microphone and then cut them in to the recording using Garage Band. You can then import this into an MP3, which makes it compatible for uploading to Buzzsprout. When I first started the podcast, I had a fancy personalised jingle I thought was really cool. However, I had to remove episodes because of copyright infringements. To avoid this, don't be fancy, just use your own voice as an intro.

3.   Ask Anyone

When I first started off, my goal was to record and publish one episode a week. I don't know why, I just did. Unbeknown to me, this was a great idea for a reason that didn't become apparent to me for some time. My first eight episodes were with friends and colleagues just chatting about them and their journey as coaches. As luck would have it, episode #9 was with Rawdon Dubois, host of one of the world's biggest fitness podcasts called "Under The Bar," episode #11 was with Dr Bob Rakowski, and episode #14 was with Christian Thibaudeau. You could say I lucked out pretty quick, but in reality, these people wouldn't have been on the show if I'd never asked.

If you'd shown me a list of the people I've interviewed when I first started, I wouldn't have believed you. Since starting in 2017 I've had (prepare for some serious name dropping now), Rawdon Dubois, Dr Bob Rakowski, Christian Thibaudeau, Paul Carter, Dave Tate, Stan Efferding, Dr Scott Steveson,

Victoria Felkar, Sebastian Oreb, Dr Stuart McGill, Dr Brian Walsh, John Meadows, and Dan Reeve on the show. I'm proud of this list but remember; they only came on the show because I asked. Out of all those people, I offered to pay every single one of them for their time. Not one of them wanted any money. I think this shows where a lot of people's hearts are really at. I would recommend always offering to pay people for their time; however, I'd say the majority will decline out of both politeness and passion for the industry. If you start a podcast and you want to have big named guests on the show, you must get over your fear of rejection and be willing for people to either say no or ignore you. Don't worry, it doesn't hurt. People will often just say they don't have time or that they're really busy. It's no reflection on you or your brand. Some people genuinely do have a lot to do and need to be smart with how they spend their time. I think the tone of your email is important as well. I'm not saying I had the perfect formula, but I always gave them a bit of a background about the show, what my goals are, and who I am. I always sent links to my website and Instagram page so they could figure me out as a person and think whether they'd like to be associated with me. I'd guess that for every one big name guest I've had on, I've had two who said no. You do the maths. What I didn't know is that iTunes has a formula. The more episodes a show has, the more it climbs the rankings. I've now started to have people contact me asking to feature on the show, which is really humbling. This has ranged from doctors in the US to TEDTalk presenters. It's exciting but all stemmed from seeing the forest through the trees and interviewing my friends in my kitchen back in 2017.

4.   Don't chase guest names, chase the quality of conversation

I know this one is a little contradictory to what I just said; however, just because someone is technically a big name doesn't mean they're going to produce good content. My goal is to provide interesting information that is applicable to the listener. If the person being interviewed doesn't provide this, then you can risk losing your audience. When looking for a guest, I always think, what would I like to hear? What would I find interesting? What would make me want to listen to more of this person? As the podcast has evolved, I've realised it's beneficial to focus on specific areas in depth rather than talk about a broad spectrum. This doesn't mean you can't digress in to different topics but it does mean the listener should be aware they're about to be educated in a specific topic to a high level. For example, a specific topic is "everything you need to know about detoxification or the female contraceptive pill or intra workout nutrition." My formula now is simple. As I have an audience, ideally I'm looking to do a 1:1 ratio of guest to solo shows. The guests don't have to be particularly well known; they just need to be a specialist in a specific area that the listener will find useful. This takes me nicely in to my last tip.

5.   Speak to one person

Although you may think it's nice to have millions of adoring fans, this is irrelevant if these people view you in a superficial way and don't actually value what you have to say. If all you are is a physique or weightlifter to someone, you're not impacting the way they conduct themselves and the quality of their life. When I do a solo podcast, my goal is to speak to one person about a problem they have. I literally talk to them, it's just a one-way conversation. As I've said many times before, one person's problem is probably many people's problem. People have so many issues but they don't vocalise or speak about because they're embarrassed or shy.

In April 2018, I was preparing for a seminar. I was going about my business in the gym one day and stumbled across some news on social media that one of my friends had died. He was thirty-five and dropped dead of a heart attack. He was one of the funniest, loveliest people you could have met and had a one-year-old son. I got in my car and on the verge of tears, recorded a podcast and called it "The most important podcast you'll ever hear." It was an extremely raw, emotional outpouring about not taking life for granted. I don't know how many listens it's had but I had one person message mc and say, "Thank you for that. I really needed to hear it and it's made me rethink a lot of things." The fact that this episode impacted a person in this way is enough for me. The hours I spent recording episodes, the money I've spent on equipment and hosting sites, it's all worthwhile when you get a message like that. That is the number one reason you should start your own show. If you resonate with one person and make them feel better that day, you've done your job.

HOW TO MAXIMISE SOCIAL MEDIA USAGE

Social media is a strange one. It's like a friend who can be really funny and great to be around but then sometimes they overstay their welcome at your house and start to get really annoying. They then start texting and calling you at 3:00am and slowly but surely you get sick of them. You think about cutting ties with this person but realise you can't as you're also in business with them and it would impact the growth of your company. I've been there. I know how you feel. In this chapter, I'll give you some useful and applicable information for maximising your social media outlets.

1.   Do the Math - How much money do you make off social media?

Let's started with finances, as this will be the one that ultimately justifies your usage of this marketing tool. To be frank, if you improve your income through using social media, it'd be pretty dumb to get rid of it. Especially as it's free. Let's use the example of an online training coach.

There a plenty of successful online coaches out there. Although the market is unregulated, there are some fantastic, hard-working trainers consistently putting out outstanding results. Say a trainer posts three times a week on Instagram. They mainly post about their clients and their results. For easy maths sake, they have a hundred clients who pay £120 a month. This works out at £12,000 divided by twelve (posts per month) and equals £1,000 per post. Now, they don't actually earn £1,000 per post passively, but they do generate £1,000 a month for their business, especially if the majority of their inquires come through Instagram. This is without doubt a valid reason for this trainer to maximise their social media platform. The problem is, I highly doubt that 90% of coaches out there earn a penny from their social media pages. We obsess about posting pictures of food, topless selfies with great lighting, and pictures in nature talking about balance, but in reality, it doesn't mean a great deal. If you don't have an online product or a passive product you can sell, spending a tonne of your time on social media isn't an effective way to run your business.

How much money does your social media make you? You could argue that the more money it generates, the more time you should be on there. If it doesn't equate to a lot, perhaps it may be a better idea to focus on your one-to-one business instead.

2.   Posting - Get in, get out

Social media is made for two types of people: the content providers and the content consumers. We all know accounts that put out awesome information constantly and we all know random account of people with fifty followers, follow 3,500 people, and have only posted seventeen pictures, half of them of their cat. That's a consumer. As trainers, your should aim to be 90% provider, 10% consumer. Don't worry if it's 80/20 at times, but generally aim to spend more time putting up your own stuff than looking at other people's. You don't have to objectively measure this, but it helps to have an idea. You'll know yourself when you're scrolling too much.

3.   Habits - Make things difficult for yourself

The biggest problem with social media is cross contamination. It's right next to all the stuff you actually need to use. I may be happily typing away with great flow and then feel a buzz in my bag. I check my What's App and answer the message, but then have a quick check of Insta to see how my post is doing. The next thing I know, five minutes have gone by and I'm six months deep into some random lifters page critiquing their deadlift 1RM max attempt. That's five minutes of writing time lost. Going on apps is purely habitual. You'll do it by default and not even notice sometimes. Make sure your social media apps are as far away from any commonly used apps on your screen set up. Don't have them on the first page and don't have them side by side to your messenger apps. You'll use them more. Think about where supermarkets put all their most decadent goods. You don't see cauliflowers being stacked up right beside the check-out till, do you? It's all chocolates and other confectionaries. Your brain and phone work in the same way. Move the chocolate to the back of the shop. Get the app as deep into your phone as possible.

4.   Maximise your page

Every now and then I catch up with my social media marketing mentor, Amy Woods. Amy started up a business called Content 10x and is amazing when it comes to everything to do with social media trends. She always gives me invaluable advice on what I should be doing with my page and how I could get more out of it. When we were discussing hashtags, she pointed out a flaw in the way I was using them. I've always thought that hashtags look needy. I thought that the more hashtags you use, the more desperate you look. She then asked me, "Are you using social media to benefit your business, or to be liked?" As mine is the former, I decided to listen to what she had to say.

Amy informed me that using commonly searched hashtags is pointless. I always assumed that using things like #fitness and #gym were great as they had 20–30 million searches under them. Wrong! It's actually the opposite. Instagram is fickle. It makes the popular people more popular and the pushes small accounts to the wayside. If you use popular hashtags, you'll be on that trend for literally a millisecond. Most posts will be spam, which will make Instagram think that you are spam. If it does this, it'll drop the amount of exposure you get. She recommended using 5–10 hashtags that have around 500,000–1,000,000 trends. This means it's popular but not so popular you won't stand a chance. Then use 5–10 hashtags with 100,000–500,000 trends with a more specific hashtag to your post, then 5–10 hashtags with REALLY specific topics to your post from anywhere between 1,000–5,000 trends. By doing this, you'll be found by people who want to find you. I hate to break it to you, but if someone types in #girlswholift, they don't want to find your page; they're looking for softcore porn. Don't waste time.

I pushed my social media ego aside and started using this method. Low and behold, followers went up, and they were real people. I check out all my new followers and they were actual legitimate accounts all similar to what I do: coaches, chiropractors, osteopaths, and doctors. There were no Russian.princess.874572836 who has no followers but instantly DMs you saying HI. Spam down, organic reach up. That's a win in my eyes. If it looks needy putting a lot of hashtags, so be it. I have passive products available online, so having actual followers does matter.

Disclaimer: Using this method will probably reduce the number of likes you get, not increase them. This may sound like a bad idea but it's only because you're getting less spam. It may be nice to see that you check Instagram and have fifty new likes. However, you need to remember these are completely irrelevant if they're not real people.

5. You be you

"Be yourself, everyone else is taken."

Another gem Amy gave me was that people gravitate towards personality, not necessarily knowledge. When assessing my online coaching page, she said that just giving away knowledge isn't really enough. People may like it, but everyone's doing that these days. It isn't enough. She recommended the 33/33/33 rule. A third of your content should be useful information. A third of your content should be the results you get or the value you provide, and a third of your content should be your personality and what you are like as a person. Being genuine online will go a long way. Don't do anything you don't feel comfortable with or things you think you should be doing because other people do it.

What your social media platform says about you?

Social media is important for personal trainers. Having a strong online presence increases your brand reputation and awareness, therefore enhancing your ability to reach more people with your services and product. It's an excellent marketing tool and this is something we should never forget. The issue for personal trainers is assuming that having a large number of followers is a necessity. It's really not, and here's why.

I can tell you now that using your following as a way of building legitimacy isn't wise. Sure, it's great to have a lot of people seeing what you do, but if gaining these followers isn't organic and systematic, you may find yourself spending a lot of time on an area that isn't generating income. In business, time is money; therefore, if you're wasting time, you're wasting money. As soon as you become emotionally attached to your online avatar, you've created a problem. Your concerns stray away from objective data and more towards the feeling of being judged and liked by people. You've blurred the lines and it's made this marketing tool into a psychological distraction. Posting content with the intention of it being liked is irrelevant. Don't get me wrong, I too enjoy the dopamine hit of opening an app and seeing a red notification flood of engagement. It does make you feel good about yourself, but here you're creating a dependency on an emotion that doesn't serve your business any use at all, unless you know how to capitalise on it. You need specifics, answers, and calls to action. You shouldn't be asking, "How can I get more likes and followers?" You should be thinking, "How can I communicate and show value to the people who I want to be working with me?" There's a big difference.

If you upload visually pleasing pictures on a regular basis at peak times with the right hashtags, your following will go up. That will work if you give it time and patience. If not, you can always buy followers if you'd like. However, people aren't dumb and having thousands of people following you and only getting a couple of dozen likes per post gives the game away. You don't want to do this as you'll lose people's respect. In my opinion, social media is all about trust. With all the information available, consumers want to see how you can help them and whether you're a reliable source. They go on your page because they find your content valuable and they ask to work with you because your product provides the answer they're looking for. Therefore, the main goal of a social media page needs to be precision and reliability.

Precision basically means taking away any form of guess work. The person visiting your page shouldn't have to figure out what you do. Rather than them thinking, "I think this person does this," you quite clearly state, "I help office workers regain their mobility." Use a demographic, use a skill, use an accomplishment; it's a clear formula. If you wanted to get stronger in the squat, bench, and deadlift, would you entertain the coach who said, "Track record for increasing elite powerlifting totals by 20 kg in six months," or would you see the guy who's bio read, "Strength and conditioning coach"? Being precise saves people time and time is your greatest foe on social media. If you lose people's attention, you lose their business.

Reliability is how consistent you are with your posting frequency, USP topic, and online persona. People will be asking themselves how much they can rely on you to give them information. If you post great content but not frequently enough, you may lose people's interest or they may believe they don't get enough from you, so unfollow you. If you deviate from one topic to another, you may look like a jack of all trades and not specific enough to one area. If you post about working with busy executives, then post a picture of you with your friends on a night out, it's not consistent with the professional theme. For me, I'm bothered about who my followers are and the information they can extract from landing on my page. I'm not too fussed about likes and the number of followers I have. I'm sure there are people with hundreds of thousands, if not millions, who don't actually monetise their market. Sure, people watch them, but they don't trust them enough to buy from them.

My goal with my social media page is for people to be able to educate themselves simply by landing on my page. Say they happened to come across my name on a train journey. They could then immerse themselves in my content and learn everything I have to say about an area. The number of likes I have per post is irrelevant; what is relevant is how much value I bring to said person through what I'm putting out. This creates fans, and fans are more likely to work with you. This is what I mean by reliability. You need to get people thinking, "I can rely on (your name) because they consistently put out great information, which I love to read. They do it on a frequent basis and I know what to expect from them."

This is where a social media schedule becomes valuable. Having a set quota of how many times you post not only allows your audience to know what to expect from you, it means you can work objectively towards a content goal. For example, you set aside one hour per week where your only goal is to make social media posts. One is a client feature, one is an exercise tutorial, one is a meal recipe. Once you have done this, you can box off social media, schedule your posts, and then focus on other tasks. If you're noticing a high level of engagement in your page, you could opt to do a live video or story a couple of times per week when you have some free time or are doing your daily commute. Be consistent and be reliable. If you do this, you'll eventually create a portfolio where your audience can see that you work with people just like them (and get results with them). They'll see that you know how to train as you upload useful tutorials and that you can provide them with meal ideas. I call this the Cookbook Theory.

Most chefs who release cookbooks have their own TV shows. You can watch them cook for free on TV, where you can extrapolate your own recipes and meal ideas. So why is it people buy their books once they hit the stores? Why do they actively opt to pay more for something they can watch for free? It's because fans want to buy things off you. They want to repay you for your free content and so are happy to purchase your products due to the level of satisfaction they've had in what you've provided. I watch Jamie Oliver's five ingredient meal programme almost every night on the Food Network (after the Bake Off, of course) yet bought his latest book as soon as it was released. I'll sometimes even sit there reading the book and watching the show. Now here's another question for you: do you think I can cook like Jamie Oliver? I'd like to think I can, but we're probably not on a par. It's the same for your audience. An amazing tutorial of you coaching a deadlift would be invaluable for a lot of people. They'll find your cues extremely useful and probably save themselves a lot of issues with their lower back. However, is this tutorial as useful as a one-to-one session with yourself? Absolutely not; you'd be able to help them tenfold in the flesh. If Jamie Oliver offered a personal cooking lesson, he'd probably be able to warrant charging thousands of pounds an hour. How busy do you think he'd be if he'd offer them for £50? You've got to think of yourself like that. How do you create fans and how do you get them to want to work with you? A lot of it is down to reliability and consistency.

IDENTIFYING YOUR AUDIENCE

If you are like me, you'll sometimes be baffled about what to put on social media. Sound too smart and you'll lose your audience; sound too dumb and people won't think you're knowledgeable. So what is the best approach and how do you really identify your target market?

The answer is, it's tricky. However, before we explore the whats and whys of content, let's first think about the so-called Instagram politics. The general trend on Instagram is that if someone follows you, you follow them back. It's a common courtesy thing: a follow for a follow. Many trainers associate having a high number of followers as being successful and so want to drive up their following without having to pay for marketing. Therefore, you follow a lot of people in the hope they follow you back. Where does that leave you? Well, most of your audience ends up being coaches and other PTs. They're not your target audience, they've just ended up being your followers by default. This is funny if you think about it. All coaches follow coaches as a means of increasing their audience but ironically this method doesn't increase their target market in the slightest. See what I'm getting at here?

If I were to go through all the people who follow me on my personal account, I'd say around 70% have a name with some sort of fitness connotation, e.g. coach, fitness, PT, training, and so on. Therefore, it's safe to assume they'll have a decent amount knowledge when it comes to training and physiology. From a marketing perspective, this isn't ideal. If you want to sell to the general population, you don't want coaches following you, you want everyday gym goers following you. These are your Smithy1990 or DannyLad23 accounts. Real people who actively use Instagram to find better ways to work out. This type of followers are gold as they're more likely to buy from you, whether it be one-to-one PT or online coaching.

Who do you want to appeal to and what do you want to grow? If you want to grow your one-to-one training business, focus on showing case studies. This includes before and after pictures, written testimonials, and video testimonials of clients posting workouts drenched in sweat. Why? So people can relate. For example, in one post you write about Dave, a forty-five-year-old who owns a business, has two kids, and wants to lose weight. You show a video of him doing a modified strongman circuit, which you can see he's finding incredibly difficult. He's pouring with sweat but loving it at the same time. At the end of the (short) clip, you put a picture of his initial photo where it's clear he's lost a couple of stone. In the write up, you talk about how it's improved his energy, confidence, and mobility levels. You use hashtags that people like Dave would search for, not the spam ones that just get you likes from fake accounts. These are things like "#Over40Training", "#Dadbod", "#DadsTraining", "#DadStrong". You've got to think, if Dave was searching for something that would suit him on Instagram, what would he type in? That's how it works.

Now, if Dave came across a picture of a muscle highlighted in green and then an in-depth analogy of the origin, insertion, and action of the muscle, he will probably lose interest quickly. He's also not likely to search for "Anatomy Education" unless he's injured. To sum up, don't just think about what the person you're looking to target is looking for. Think about how they'd find you as well. How would you gain their interest? Imagine if you posted about your current client base over and over and your followers increased with an audience that consisted of virtually the exact same avatar you've been posting about. Happy days! This is the holy grail of business development and marketing. If all your audience falls in to your "buyer's market," you'll have a much better chance of getting busy.

Let's look at the world of online training. First, who is online training for and who does it suit the best? This to me is simple: young gym goers. If someone goes to the gym, is between the age of 18–30 and uses Instagram, they fall into a pretty decent demographic to target for online coaching. The only issue is, online coaching is becoming even more saturated that one-to-one PT and it's even more unregulated (which is scary). If you use a visually orientated social media outlet, your posts need to be visually pleasing. Most of the audience will be attracted to trainers who are really ripped, big, or strong. If this is your audience, you have to play the game on aesthetics and post visual before and afters, pictures of yourself, and images that show you're legit. From a business point of view, I'd rather be the guy with 100,000 followers looking to build an online business than the guy with 1,000 followers. To get these followers, you either need to play the game or be patient. The game isn't always the most integral or morally fulfilling one though. My point is, you can't get annoyed with Instagram just because *you* think your content is good, but nobody is seeing it. I'm sure that your content is excellent but it's not going to get seen if you don't play the game. A visual outlet needs visual means and unless your posts are exceptionally good or The Rock gives you a shout out, you will always be left frustrated with your efforts to rewards ratio. Remember the golden rule:

High following + Same type of follower = Greater Inquiry/ Product Uptake (given you have a product)

Putting educational content on Instagram isn't the most efficient way of using this social media platform. Not that many people are going to pay attention to it. Why? Well, because if you go too advanced, the people who find your content useful are other coaches. They may comment with "great post" or "well explained" but that's probably not going to increase the likelihood of them working with you. If they know what you're on about it's because they likely attended the same course you did. I'm not saying you shouldn't do educational posts online, far from it. I just want you to understand that it may not be the best way of driving up numbers to increase revenue. I used to spend three or more hours a week recording YouTube videos and putting them online for free. They got great feedback but made me zero money. From a business perspective, it made no financial sense at all. Just remember, time is money and social media is just a part of your business, not your entire business. How you come across online is irrelevant if you're not making a decent living in real life. If you feel you want to educate people then please, feel free to do so. Just don't be tempted into thinking sounding smart online will boost your business. Being authentic online will. People will like you more if you're honest about your current levels of knowledge rather than trying to be something you're not.

Most of your content should reflect the product you wish to sell the most. You should have an avatar (ideal client) you wish to sell to at the forefront of your mind. Speak to this person and post things that they would find useful. Then, most importantly, be consistent with it. If you go from biomechanics, to microbiome, to strength periodisation, to psychology, all of which are covered in PhD-like format, people won't know what to expect from you. If you do two client features showing a real-life case study and one evening meal recipe of your page per week, people will be able to see how you can help them. Do it consistently for six months and see how your market expands.

Once you've built an online brand through consistency and speaking to the right demographic, you then need to have an accessible means of your market interacting and working with you. This needs to be as simple and efficient as possible. One of the biggest mistakes I made was assuming that just because people thought you had great content, they'd flock to working with you. This isn't the case. People may inquire, but unless you provide fool-proof ways of contacting about your services, don't expect to be inundated with leads. Simplicity wins, and here's why.

A lot of people worry about being too pushy with their marketing strategy online. I fell into this bracket and would never actively advertised my online training services on social media. This was purely out of stubbornness and not wanting to seem needy. However, things changed once I set up an online training business, which heavily relied on lead generation via social media. You have to think of it like this. You're flicking through your Instagram feed after typing in #Burger and find a restaurant that looks like it serves great food. You see a burger that tickles your fancy and so immediately have gaged interest. You and your partner are looking for a place to go out this weekend and so are in the market for a meal out. You scroll through the page and are now certain you want to eat at this place. There's a problem though: there's no link to where the restaurant is, how you get to it, or how much the burger costs. You click on the website and this information is still hard to come by. To find out more, you'd have to message them directly and say, "Hey, I live in X town, do you have any of your restaurants near me?" The reality is you're unlikely to do this. You'd likely scroll on and find an equally appetising burger where you know where you can find it. The first burger place didn't try to sell to you, so you didn't buy. If that same burger place had had a button in its bio that took you straight to the book a table link, you'd be booked in for your Friday night feast in an instant. The call to action was too vague and difficult, so they lost your custom. If you want people to work with you online, you need to make your services clear and precise for them to see. You also want to reduce any form of resistance possible when it comes to inquiring about your services. If you can help people, make sure you tell them regularly about how you can do this.

I appreciate that the online market is saturated and fickle. However, if a burger joint uploaded regular pictures of mouth-watering concoctions coupled with a restaurant brimmed to the rafters with happy customers, it becomes a no brainer. If you feature happy clients who get results on a regular basis and emphasise how you can help them, people will inquire. There's a big difference between this and the people who proclaim to have the best burgers in town yet post no pictures of their product or restaurant. If you're doing a good job, you need to let people know about it. The old call to action used to be email, but I believe someone following you on social media is as good as having their email address. Emails are likely to fall into spam and not be read. You can guarantee that most people will check their social media at some point in the day. Although a click funnel to getting people's email is advisable, I wouldn't say it's the be all and end all. Instead, direct them to your web page, where you explain pricing, packages, what to expect, and what happens subject to payment. You need to have something that is readily available and answers all their questions. I've done email campaigns where I've released several free PDFs including recipe books and workout plans. I built up an email list of a couple of hundred names, but then had the issue of writing out regular email to them to keep them engaged. My workload was going up but for little gain. I do think that social media has made this step unnecessary, so it wouldn't be at the forefront of my priorities. I'm sure some people have had incredibly success from this; however, if you can direct someone to your website direct from a social media outlet, it cuts out the middle man.

The best call to action is the one that makes the potential client feel like they're in the safest hands. If you sell too aggressively, you may put them off. If you don't sell quickly enough, you may miss their custom. In my opinion, it all comes down to experience and getting a feel for what they person needs and what their agenda is. As this is the case, I would offer to have a quick chat with potential clients (both online and offline) so that you can disarm them and get a feel for their personality. If they opt for the call, you know they're expressing decent interest. If they don't, you know they fall into the category of a cold lead. Approach all your calls with one objective: to explain the value you provide. Be as honest as possible and if the person doesn't choose to use your services, it's only 5–10 minutes of your time gone. A little goes a long way. A small phone call could lead to a client who spends hundreds of pounds with you over the course of years. Building rapport is essential and a phone call does this much faster than any email.

ONLINE TRAINING

Online training is one of the most misunderstood areas of the industry. It's something that can supplement your income and business if done correctly and not something you have to do because everyone else is. If you use it smartly, you can build a flexible lifestyle that accommodates you and your family. This being said, I never recommend totally losing touch with the gym floor as this takes away a critical skill needed to be an excellent coach: personal observation. This section is all about how to build an online training profile in tandem with your one-to-one coaching business.

How does the following situation sound to you? You wake up at 5:00am, meditate for ten minutes, eat, get changed, write your goals down for the day, and set off for work at 5:45am. You get to work for 6:10am with enough time to prepare for your client and make a coffee before your first session. You do three clients back to back from 6:30–9:30, then have a half hour break for something to eat. You have a further two clients from 10:00–12:00 before getting ready and training for a couple of hours from 12:30–2:30. Your working day at the gym finishes at 3:00pm. Once home, you chill out, have a shower, then spend from 3:30-5:00pm doing online check-ins for five clients via email. You spend around twenty minutes per check in, addressing food, training, and any problems the client may have. This is what you do five days per week, Monday to

Friday. You don't work past 12:00pm in the gym and don't work past 5:00pm at home. Who would like this situation? Sound realistic? I can tell you for certain that it is.

The way I see it, you don't need hundreds of clients to have a successful online business. Having 10–15 online clients paying double your hourly rate per month is the perfect and most manageable supplementary income for your one-to-one coaching. Here are my top tips on how to run an online business.

1.   Specify your target market

If you're a strongman, train strongmen. If you're a runner, train runners. If you're a post-natal mum wanting to strengthen her core after giving birth… you get my point. One thing I wouldn't advise doing is taking on every Tom, Dick, and Harry who inquire for your services. The money may seem tempting, but you'll quickly get frustrated. Consider this example:

You charge £80 a month for online coaching. If people pay for three months upfront, they get it for £225 (monthly rate £75). Rather than specifying who your services are for, you simply say, "Available for all people of all capabilities." The more inquires the better, right? This will be to your detriment for two reasons. First, how do people know if you're for them? How do they know that you can fix their specific problems? How do they know that you've done it with people just like them in the past? The answer is, they don't. If you want really good Chinese food, you go to a quaint, bespoke Chinese restaurant. You don't go to your local Beefeater and order from the Chinese side of the menu. Specificity wins. Your social media should follow similar topics with anomalies every now and then. It's okay if 20% of your client base doesn't fit your exact model, but try to have a common theme. For example, for performance athletes, talking about performance markers, performance enhancement, and performance mindset is important. It's unlikely someone will contact you for a "twelve-week transformation" but this is perfect because they're not the people you want to work with. Second, when you take on an array of clientele, you get an array of different needs and expectations. Working with a housewife whose nutritional education comes from *Hello* magazine and *Loose Women* is extremely different to working with a twenty-four-year-old office worker who loves bodybuilding. Both of these people may be paying ~£75 a month but trust me, the work you put in won't be the same. With the young bodybuilder, you may send her programme, macros, and dietary changes once per week and have perfect compliance. She is robotic and loves to process, knows how to train, and trains hard. Your check-ins take ten minutes max and you get an easy ride for your £75 a month. She is essentially your perfect client.

The mum of two, on the other hand, still can't get her head around macros. She feels like you've given her too much food and doesn't understand the importance of weighing out her food instead of just cutting carbs. She questions all your methods and rather than sending health marker information during her check-in, it's a long-winded email about social events, the challenges of having the kids, and getting annoyed as to why she hasn't lost any weight. You want to ensure you give her the best service possible, so send a detailed reply to every email. You are professional and understanding in your approach but unfortunately this is time consuming. She replies back and you get into an email conversation. This interaction takes up nearly two hours of your week.

Here you have two people who produce very different outcomes. Your young bodybuilder will be low maintenance, compliant, and a great advert for future clientele. The working mum will be high maintenance, hard work, and probably won't achieve the results she wants. Which one do you think you should try to attract? This isn't me saying that you'll never get a result with people like this. Sometimes small tweaks can go a long way with certain clientele. However, a thorough screening is essential when it comes to taking on a client. Asking things like, "Have you counted calories before?", "What has worked well for you in the past?", "What are your current nutritional beliefs" are key as you are starting to get a picture of what this person is like. Just like one-to-one training, you need to create your perfect client.

This is where a phone call can become invaluable prior to someone working with you. Although it is your job to highlight why they should work with you, you also must be integral and explain if you're not for them as well. Imagine that someone said, "I'm good with my diet and am happy with what I weigh, I'm just unsure as to whether I'm doing certain exercises right." If this person were based five hours away from you, you'd have to explain that seeing an in-person PT would be much more beneficial for them. Desperation is the thief of integrity. Don't see every phone call as a sale. If you don't believe you can help someone to meet their needs, you shouldn't sign them up.

2.   Do more than others (health markers, digestion, sleep)

We've established that you need to find the right audience for your services. Now we need to look into what services you provide. A simple way to improve your business is to find out what the competition is doing and do it better. This sounds brutal, but it's true. A typical online plan includes a training programme, macronutrient guide, and weekly check-ins. It's safe to say that if you don't do these, you're not truly an online coach, just a person who gives out programmes on the internet. You're not coaching, you're providing information. To make a successful living out of doing just these three commodities, you'd either need to have a large social media following or be extremely good at writing programmes and changing macros. I'm not saying the latter isn't possible, but the reality is you'll require the former if you're going to attract a lot of people. Unfortunately, people are fickle. More of a following makes you seem more legitimate in what you do. If you have a modest audience and take pride in your work, you need to go above and beyond to create a service that trumps your competitors. So, how do you do that?

My first recommendation is to look at the big picture. Are you taking into consideration all the variables that play a part in your client getting results? These include sleep, digestion, stress, lifestyle, training quality, and energy expenditure. You have to piece together the puzzle and show the person that you care about their wellbeing. Demonstrate that you know how to explain plateaus or lack of results. If someone just gets a programme from you, what do you discuss during the check-in? "How's the programme going?" This isn't exactly professional, is it? However, if someone fills out a form that shows their sleep has been really poor that week and training performance has suffered, this is what you address during the check-in. You give them a list of all the things they can do to improve their sleep and make sure it's back on track by the next week. This is coaching. Teaching people how to modify their diet, training, and lifestyle to get results whilst following your plan. What I like to do is create a spreadsheet with all these features on them. Each week I download the client's check-in and then figure out the averages for that week—average steps, average waking heart rate, average stool quality (yep, you read that correctly). Then I can assess how they're progressing from week to week. It's great when somebody loses weight over a twelve-week period; however, it's even better when they lose weight, improve sleep, reduce stress, have better digestion, and move more. If you have recorded all the subjective data, it's a fantastic way to show the client their progress from week 1 to 12. Imagine this as a marketing tool on your website and social media:

"Debbie started with me back in January stating she wanted to lose a stone. She has a stressful job and works long hours and very much struggles to get restful sleep. In the past sixteen weeks she has improved sleep duration by an average of one hour, with subjective sleep quality increasing by 25%. As a by-product, Debbie's average waking heart rate has dropped by 15 bpm, indicating a physiological drop in stress. During this time Debbie has lost 10kg and is delighted with her progress. She has more energy, confidence, but above all else, dramatically improved health markers."

You could combine this a before and after picture of Debbie, along with a graph to show her stats. Now, who are you more likely to choose? The person who uploads posts like this or the person who brashly proclaims, "it's just calories in vs calories out, it's not that hard people"? What's amazing is that all these tracking tools are now readily available for the general population. We can easily track sleep, heart rate, blood glucose, recovery, expenditure, and so on in extremely easy ways. If you incorporate these factors into your online training, it'll show that you go above and beyond the competition to provide the best service possible.

3.   Cater for the individual

With my online coaching, my business partner and I devised a questionnaire for each client prior to starting. We look at their age, job, situation, lifestyle, training experience, and goals and then see which feedback markers are the most applicable. This helps trim a lot of fat and know what will work. For example, if the person is in their twenties, active on Instagram, works as a personal trainer, and has a supportive partner, we can assume they'll be accustomed to macros, tracking, health markers, and so on. Therefore, we can look at all these aspects and ask them to track them. If the person is in their forties, has an office job, has never been to the gym before, and doesn't follow industry leaders on social media, we may have to adapt their approach. Waking up and doing blood glucose levels, HRV, and taking ten supplements before having steak and eggs isn't realistic for a working dad of three. Look at their situation and say to this guy, "Track how many steps you do and how many calories you eat a day. Then send over your weight every Friday morning after taking it at the same time in the same place." Rather than having to fill in a NASA style spreadsheet, all this person has to do is track weight, expenditure, and calories. For this person's initial 6–8 weeks, this will be sufficient. This isn't to say a parent or office worker shouldn't track all their variables. In your questionnaire, you could ask the following: Which one of these health markers are you familiar with or have tracked before? Then list the variables you like to measure. You can then tell them you'd like them to track what they are familiar with so you don't encounter any resistance or confusion. In the meantime, you could send over your pre-written PDF with an explanation of why they should be tracking those variables. If a situation occurs where introducing a new variable to track would be useful, it's your job to coach and explain why they should be tracking said commodity.

"I'd like you to start taking morning blood glucose. You do this by doing X, Y, and Z. We're doing this because I would like to increase carbs in your next training phase but first we need to make sure your insulin sensitivity is where it should be. Otherwise, the carbs may not be used efficiently. To learn more about insulin and carbs, read pages 10–20 of our training manual."

It's not realistic for 100% of your clients to be 100% compliant. However, this doesn't mean you can't try to get them to be. Either screen your clients initially, be picky, and only take on golden nuggets, or adapt your services so that you increase the likelihood of them tracking the variables you want to see.

4.   Create a community

People like to belong to things. As simple as it sounds, I believe it's a primal instinct to want to be part of a group. There's safety in numbers and being part of a tribe provides a sense of security and guidance. Just like fully grown men wear replica jerseys of their favourite football team and women sport handbags made by their favourite fashion designer, when you're proud of the community you belong to, you want to show the world. How many of you right now are wearing some form of clothing that indicates you are part of a group? To create a community, you need to do two things: first, find an easily accessible portal for people to communicate, and second, have a specific theme or goal that people discuss on a regular basis. If you want to get good at something, look at the common denominators from the people who do things at the forefront of their industry. They haven't got there by accident. I appreciate you may feel a bit like a prima donna for painting yourself as a guru and leader. However, it all comes down to the way you present yourself and how you communicate to people.

So how do you go about it? The simplest way to create a community these days is to set up a Facebook group. Get all your clients to join the group and then you can post regularly and get people to interact. When I used to do group training, I would see a direct correlation between the number of times people posted their meals in the online groups and how much weight they lost. Honestly, the more people uploaded, the more they seemed to lose. I used to say, "A post for a pound." This makes perfect sense if you think about it. By regularly interacting, people remind themselves they are part of a group, have a goal, and need to stay on track. It also creates the important psychological aspect of maintaining a streak. Once you've posted 5–6 meals in a row, you create a run. Once this run picks up momentum, you don't want to break it. This is an excellent way of creating accountability. What's also great about a group is that you can address specific questions in one area. I can guarantee that during a weight loss phase, a group of people will have the same questions and queries as each other. Rather than typing out the same answer over and over, you can answer the question in a communal setting so everyone can see. As you also have the added benefit of the comments section, you can then go into further detail in an interactive manner. This creates incredibly value for the clients.

If you're working with the general population for fat loss, one of the biggest obstacles you'll encounter is something I've coined Dietary Fatigue. This is when you get bored of eating the same thing over and over again. My solution is to get good at cooking the same thing; however, since you can't guarantee everyone will have culinary competency, it helps when you can add easy to make meal varieties to the group that everyone can see. On occasion, you'll get a really zealous client who'll upload recipes themselves for the group. This is awesome as your own client base is now subsidising your content. How good is that? You want people to interact, you want people to have banter, you want people to get to make online friends in your group. If you promote this, you create a tribe where you're the leader. It has nothing to do with status or ego, it's purely just that you were the instigator of the group. People are more likely to stay with you for longer if they have a feeling of belonging. Also think of it as passive income. Okay, maybe not passive, but it means you could add more value to your product for the same amount of work.

Let's say someone pays £80 per month for your online services. They get a programme from you, diet plan, and check-in once per week. This is a great service that I'm sure you could validate if we broke it down. Let's say you have a Facebook group in which you religiously post in twice per day. You upload exercises, recipes, motivational quotes, links to useful resources, meal pics, etc. Now every time this person checks their social media, there you are. At 7:00am your breakfast pic says, "What's everyone else having?" At lunch time, it's a video of your training session saying, "What's everyone else training today?" At the evening meal, add a picture saying, "How is everyone else winding down this evening?" If you upload three per day for let's say a total communication time of five minutes, the person now gets a perceived interaction of two hours per week. Five minutes x 21 (3 post 7 times a week) = 105 minutes + 15 minute check in = 120 minutes. Monthly time investment: 8 hours. Their perceived hourly rate: £10 per hour. Now, it obviously doesn't work exactly like this and providing a break-down of this nature to your clients themselves wouldn't be advisable. However, being interactive with your own Facebook group will (subconsciously) massively improve your clients perception of value for your services. If they don't continue with you and you remove them from the group (which you should) they then miss their morning motivation, daily recipes, and live Q & A's.

Your online reputation is just as important as your in-person reputation. Just because social media is the most commonly used method of generating online client leads, this doesn't mean you still won't get customers from word of mouth referrals. Brand standards are essential. Here's what I recommend doing to maintain the best online coaching customer service possible.

One of the main things I took away from interviewing John Meadows was how much work ethic comes in to play with online coaching. I think the biggest fallacy when it comes to the online training is that it creates this laptop, entrepreneurial lifestyle where you can earn a tonne of money by sending a few emails a week. The reality is this isn't true at all. The guys who earn the big bucks in the online training world have to work for every penny. Eight hours of online work a day for seven days a week. It's an unrelenting schedule of constantly checking in with clients whilst maintaining the highest standard. They don't get there by accident. When John Meadows was in his online training peak (circa 2012) he worked up to having 250 online clients at one time. He said that he could have completed all his emails and be up to date with everything, go for lunch for an hour, and come back to sixty unread emails. He said that his policy, no matter what, was to reply to a client within twenty-four hours. This explains why you only get 1–2 sentence replies whenever you email him. Now, you could say that it's easy for someone like John Meadows to get busy, as he's John Meadows, one of the most famous bodybuilders in the world. This is true, but there are a lot of people out there with a high-profile following who I doubt are bringing in what he was a month. Having more followers doesn't always mean earning more money, but having an excellent product or service that people want to use does. Be hell bent on providing the best customer service possible. Doing the basics well is all you need to initially focus on. Remember, 10–15 clients allows you to hit that sweet spot of income where your gym rent can be covered from your laptop. Here are some tips on maintaining professionalism for online training.

1.   Let them know your schedule

You can't get frustrated at people if they don't know where they stand. If a client is constantly messaging you and you're getting annoyed, maybe it'd have been in your best of interests to tell them at the beginning how your services work. Explain your hours, when you reply to emails, and what to expect. If you do it in a polite, tactful way, they'll understand your reasoning. I do my one-to-one sessions between 7:00am and 1:30pm. I don't like to work past 6/7:00pm, so I try to get all my work done as early as possible. If I get a cancellation during the morning, the first thing I do is answer emails. Explaining to online (and one-to-one) clients when you work isn't egotistical or arrogant, it's practical. It shows you're in control of your schedule and not sporadic with your time. Again, the best thing to do would be to write a PDF and send it through to the client as part of a welcome pack.

2.   Give them reply time expectations

This such a simple thing to maximise that goes a long way. One of my biggest pet peeves is a poor reply time. A couple of days is acceptable, but over 5–7 days is an absolute joke. With online clients, try to reply to all emails or messages in some format within twenty-four hours. If you're mad busy and rushed off your feet, simply send a one sentence message saying, "Hi, just acknowledging I've seen your email and will reply tomorrow afternoon after my morning sessions." After doing this, the first thing I do is make a note on my to-do list to message this person when I next sit down to do laptop work. I will hold my hands up and say I've done this before then totally forgot to email the person. They'll usually politely send a reminder, but it doesn't look great. Being thorough and prompt with your check-in responses will do much more for your online business than hundreds of likes and followers. Trust me. Be integral and do things right. It is tit for tat though. If you get a busy exec or Houdini who takes 4–5 days to get back to you, don't break your back to reply to them immediately. I'd obviously reply within twenty-four hours, but people do need to see that the more effort they put in to you, the more effort you put in to them.

3.   Charge More for What's App/Messenger Support

You're not just a personal trainer. You may be a husband, wife, boyfriend, girlfriend, musician, artist, chef, you name it. You do have a life outside personal training. One-to-one clients pay you several hundreds of pounds a month for your services and require a good level of customer service by default. However, it's not acceptable to get a message saying, "I'm just out shopping now and they're out of mackerel. What other type of fish should I get?" from an online client at 9:00pm whilst I'm winding down with my wife. Some people massively take liberties and see you as a slave, not a coach. For every golden nugget who is a perfect angel when it comes to check-ins and compliancy, you can get one person who thinks you should be at their beck and call 24/7. If these people want to contact you regularly, they need to be paying more. One of the questions we ask on our online training questionnaire is, "If I was unsure about something on my plan I would…" Followed by 4–5 options. This gives us a good indication as to what this person is like and how much assistance they need. If they answer, "contact my coach immediately," explain to them that type of service requires an upgrade. It's not because you don't want to help, it's to protect your own free time with family, which is precious. The person will either pay you more (which is good for you) or figure things out themselves. A lot of the questions probably can wait until their next email check in or simply be posted in the Facebook group.

There are exceptions to the rules when clients have competitions or shows coming up. If I'm working with a strength athlete, I'd want to see absolutely all their main lifts every session. A strength athlete is different to a general population body comp client though. If I get sent a video of a squat or deadlift in the evening, I'm happy to watch it or at least reply to it first thing in the morning. What you don't want is for people to think you're constantly at the end of the phone whilst they're out doing their weekly shop. Set standards, set guidelines, set expectations. Let all your online clients know where they stand and what to expect from you and you'll have a much more successful, efficient business.

How to Subsidise Your Gym Rent with an Online Business

Do you ever worry about paying your gym rent? Does it loom over you every month so that you can't relax about finances? What if there was a way to make all your one-to-one PT sessions profit? Your gym rent could be completely subsidised by doing laptop work from anywhere, anytime. Here is a simple strategy that went extremely well for me at every independent gym I worked in.

The issue with generating leads online is that these people don't know you. To get to know you, they need to watch or read your content for a long time. When you talk to someone in person, you get a feel for their mannerisms, nature, and energy. It's easy and instinctive to figure out if you like someone after an initial personal interaction. This will dictate whether you want to do business with them. When first starting up your online business, don't go looking for clients all over the internet, look for people right there in front of you in the gym where you work. Every single person who goes to a gym could do with a personal trainer—remember that. The two biggest obstacles you'll face are the value people see in a trainer and the price. Once these are broken, uptake in your product is a logical decision. Follow this step by step guide and not only will you not have to worry about your monthly gym rent, you'll also be able to readjust your working hours to suit you better.

Step 1 - Identify

How much do you need to earn? People think that online training means having 50–100 clients these days. This creates an element of learned helplessness as you feel like you don't know where to start. My advice is to find out what you'd be comfortable charging. The reason is that selling something that is under-priced is extremely easy. Imagine trying to sell one personal training session on the high street for £1,000. You could interact with hundreds of people and would be extremely lucky to get a bite. Now imagine trying to sell a Ferrari Enzo for £1,000 in the same scenario. You'd be able to sell that extremely quickly. Why? High value, low price. First figure out what you would be comfortable to sell. If someone asked you the price, you could confidently say how much it was per month and not sweat at all. This will be personal to you; however, I wouldn't recommend every going lower than £50 a month. If it's too cheap, people won't see any value in it at all.

Step 2 - Calculate

As you now know you're online training rate, all you do now is set a goal of covering your gym rent with this product. This is so regardless of quiet or busy months for your one-to-one service, you'll always have a residual income to fall back on. Once you divide your gym rent by your monthly online coaching fees, you have a target. Quite simply, £500/£50 equals ten online clients.

Step 3 - Plan

An uptake and retention rate of two people per month means that in five months' time, your rent will be subsidised. You will no longer have to worry about making rent each month and you can do this during your down time at work. Once you've hit this target, you could drop clients who train at times you don't like. If you use this method when working at a commercial gym, you could drop gym shifts or classes, or again, afford to drop clients who don't fit in with your schedule. It's totally possible for you to work the hours you want in six months' time.

Step 4 - Interact

When it comes to interacting with people, don't think of it as being able to sell to everyone to you; view it as being able to help everyone you see. Taking money from people isn't a bad thing. Your services remove the guess work for people, gives them accountability, but most of all ensures they're not doing anything in the gym that is potentially dangerous. Welcome any type of interaction in any format, get to know people, and offer your help at any chance you get. The biggest apprehension anyone will have with a trainer is worrying about them selling they services. It's why people in the gym avoid interactions. If your product is reasonably priced, this fear is removed.

Step 5 - Growth

Once you have hit your target, you are then in a commanding position. You can either cap your in-person online PT intake, creating a waiting list, or you could increase fees by £5 per month to generate more money per unit. Once your gym rent is covered, I then move on to reworking your schedule and say to clients who train at times you don't want to work anymore that your hours have changed. You can validate doing this because your gym rent is covered.

Don't ever be afraid of offering impromptu extra value for your in-person online clients. A little goes a long way and putting on a monthly class or workshop exclusively for them creates a tremendous amount of value. The more they talk about you, the better. You can offer them one-off PT sessions at a discounted rate or simply push them towards just doing one session per month. The main thing is you create an in-person following in your gym who allow you to have flexibility and financial peace of mind.

THE 5 X 5 RULE FOR DEVELOPMENT

One of my biggest objectives with The 5 x 5 Rule isn't to lay out a specific guide you need to follow. This would be naive of me as every coach has their own niche, speciality, and goals. I don't want to simply teach you what I've done, but rather highlight a thought process whereby you can design your own blueprint. With The 5 x 5 Rule for development, we first need to reverse engineer the situation you'd like to be in, then work backwards following a specific and measurable plan. It'd be easy for me to tell you to write a to-do list, learn some muscles, meditate, post on social media, and interact with people, but how well would this suffice on Dragon's Den? You need rules to follow that mean you'll develop, your finances will improve, and that mean you never forget what your job's purpose is: to improve the lives of others.

Business is about finding the right balance between delayed gratification and enough return to get you through your initial phases. Focus too much on the future and you may lose sight of what matters here and now; focus too much on your current situation and you never build for the future. This is a skill you need to work on constantly. It's all well and good wanting to earn £10,000 a month in five years' time, but it doesn't mean a great deal if you're not currently earning enough money to cover your basic expenses. To build a successful business, you need to first have systems in place to comfortably break even, then look to build your brand. A practical example of this is consolidating all your current business into a monthly wage. Get all your existing clients on to a monthly direct debit worth £2,000 a month. If your outgoings are £1,250 a month, you are now in a position to build. If you haven't done this, podcasts, articles, and a booming social media presence must wait. You must do the basics first because business development requires a hell of a lot of unpaid work and even more faith in your own return. Take this book for example. If I've dedicated around 500 hours to writing, reading, and editing this project, that's a significant amount of time I've lost doing other things that could have been actively earning me money. If I wasn't first comfortable and had a consistent income, writing this book would have either been a bad business move or one hell of a gamble.

Rule 1 of Development

Development, defined as personal growth or substantial investment in to building your brand, is only warranted once you have established a solid foundation of income through training people or gym shifts. A foundation is classed as delivering enough sessions to earn 1.5 times that of your average outgoings. Do not make your life unnecessarily difficult. You must earn the right to develop and this must come from solidifying a routine where your income is consistent. Gym floor hours and classes are perfectly acceptable initially. Do not be afraid to do your time in the industry.

Despite rule number 1 seeming obvious for new trainers, several coaches who have been in the industry for a significant time still don't abide by it. They may be earning a decent wage and they may be building their brand; however, their development is being stifled by a misperception of growth coming from poorly measured commodities. Being a well-educated, professional coach who is passionate means nothing from a financial perspective. Although I highly recommend all coaches to conduct themselves in this manner, I know a lot of people who do not capitalise on their knowledge and do not invest with a mindset of direct return. Remember, you can't tell people that you're clever. You are only smart in the eye of the client. A client may think you are smart if you change the setup of an exercise to accommodate for an injury or if you know there are four calories in one gram of protein. "Smart" is an unregulated term in the fitness industry. It's subjective. If you don't have clients and you're not where you want to be financially, the time invested into your education becomes in vain.

Rule 2 of Development

Before embarking on an educational course, seminar, or certification, first factor in how long it will take you to recuperate your money. This comes from writing anything from a 3–12-month business model factoring in how you make a return of your investment plus interest. This will not only get you to select your educational materials more wisely, it will prompt you to think more like a business. For example, you select an online course that costs £600 for the year. You know you will finish your course by month six of your financial year. Eight weeks prior to finishing your course, you inform your current client base that your hourly rate will be increasing by £1.50 per hour. If you do this, you will have regained your initial investment plus 20% interest in six-months, given you are consistently delivering twenty sessions per week. All investments into development must yield a return that you could not have already gained in your existing business. If they don't, they aren't worth investing in.

Rule 2 may sound surprising given that I'm a huge advocate of learning anatomy and constant development. I'd like to reiterate that investment into education and studying are two separate commodities. You should always be studying in some format and I am by no means saying education should be put on a back burner. I just want to ensure that your income is always protected and that you don't get a false sense of security by thinking that investing in education is the answer. I was guilty of this for years. CPD does not equate to more earnings.

Ultimately, the only factor that impacts how much your charge is your own ability to ask confidently for more money. If you want to invest in your education, I strongly recommend doing it in a field that you love and not a field that you're unsure of or think you should know. Work on your passion, as this will come easiest for you to learn.

Another factor you may have overlooked is asking your client base straight up what would make their sessions more valuable. Whether it be by email or in person, periodically send your clients feedback forms or surveys asking for constructive feedback on how you could do better. You could even send a list of the courses you are considering doing and ask your client base which one they would benefit them the most. If they have no idea what they are, just put them in layman's terms: one to ease joint pain over time, one for calculating diet plans, and so forth. You want to create happy clients because a strong word of mouth referral business is worth more than thousands of online followers for a personal trainer. This is what we're forgetting. Your current client base is your most valuable resource. Use this to base your development from. It's also a good way to get critical feedback. Remember, you can't be precious or protective when something is simply not up to par. Bias to your own services is extremely unwise.

Rule 3 of Development

Constantly review your clients' experience and what they receive from you. Give yourself performance reviews from your clients and never forget that they are always your number one priority. Whether it be in person or online, customer service should always be your primary agenda—not followers, not popularity, not anything subjective and disposable. Saying to investors that your business has a five-star average rating on Trust Pilot and you haven't had to spend a penny on marketing in the past year due to word of mouth referrals is invaluable. Make this your goal in business. Ask clients for an unbiased, critical review of how you can get better, then take the information on board and apply it. Remember that there is a market for people who will always have personal trainers. They will always want someone there to train them and it might as well be you. They will welcome paying that little bit extra if they know that they're in safe hands. Long term clients will stay with you throughout price increases if they can see your investment has directly benefited them.

"Jump and the net will appear." Really think about that quote for a second. All the self-development in the world is irrelevant if you don't work on your own belief systems. I wanted to leave as much metaphysical methods out of this book as possible because they are impractical if you don't believe them yourself. I've read a plethora of self-help books and admit it can be frustrating when they simply state, "you need to change your mindset." This is as vague as it is helpful. You couldn't turn up on Dragon's Den and say, "I believe in myself." It's not factual, it's not objective, and takings someone's word for something doesn't suffice in business. If you have a belief system, you can't think it, you must be it.

The fact of the matter is, your fees will never change unless you change them yourself. It's easy to convince yourself that you're doing all the right things to move forward in business, but ultimately your income will never increase unless you make bold, uncomfortable actions to improve it. Your business will only develop as your mindset develops. A change in mindset comes from constantly reiterating to yourself your worth and the minimum you'd accept to earn per hour. Just like it's important to be critical of your progress, you must also praise yourself and appreciate how far you've come. If clients are happy and get results, and if you are professional, thorough, and provide a great service, you must value yourself. Growth in the world of the self-employed relies heavily on self-efficacy. You need to ensure you truly believe you deserve the money you want and then you need to ask for it. Jump and the net will appear means doing the unknown and having faith that it will pay off. Once you have broken this barrier, it becomes a natural process. You'll only accept a certain fee per hour, which will grow with your business.

Rule 4 of Development
You are only worth what you believe you're worth. You can educate yourself all you want, but the true value of your time and business lies in

*the value you see in yourself. Working on mindset is quite a vague term;
however, quantifying your time as a set value isn't. You must always
consider what one hour of your time is worth. Measure this based on your
experience, knowledge, results, client feedback, effort, and thirst to
improve. When you add everything up, you start to see the true value in
yourself. Increasing your fees isn't just about money; it's about your own
inner dialogue and self-esteem. You need to believe it before any paying
customer will believe it. If it helps to write it down in present tense, then
do so. Repeatedly writing what you want to be charging so that you see it
every day is an excellent way of reiterating to yourself your dedication to
move forward. If you do this, plus abide by the other rules, charging more
will just seem logical rather than scary.*

The reason establishing your own hourly rate is so important
is because time literally equates to money in service-based jobs.
No matter how much you increase your fees in your years as a
trainer, your limiting factor will always be that you exchange
time for money. You sell a service, not a product, and the
ability to expand a service always boils down to being able to
replicate the USP service given by the initial supplier. The
other area we need to look at is potential for volume. As your
time to deliver sessions is limited, the only other variable that
can be manipulated is price. This is the opposite to the way
conventional, scalable businesses work. Think of it like this:
would you rather sell coffee for £2.50 a cup or work as a
personal trainer for £50 an hour? It sounds like a bizarre
proposal but look at the situation from a business perspective.
Don't make a hasty decision too quickly; first do the maths.

Say you're selling coffee for £2.50 per unit on average. You
have other products such as lattes, espressos, and teas, but your
average spend per customer is £2.50. Once everything has
been accounted for, such as rent on your shop, outgoings, and
products, your net profit per unit sold is £1.50. Now let's look
at the personal trainer. They charge £50 per hour; however,
from this you must subtract the cost of working at the gym
they're in (which will fluctuate depending on session delivery),
travel expenses, educational fees, monthly subscriptions, and so
forth. These are all the things that contribute to running their

business. Their net profit per unit sold ends up at £35 per hour. Seems like a no-brainer, right? You'd obviously go for the one-to-one trainer's job. It pays over twenty-three times per unit sold. It seems logical, but it's only half of the equation. An equally important factor is your ability to sell something in volume and how much you are involved in the process. If a coffee shop can sell sixty units an hour in its busiest times during 6:00-9:00am, this means a net profit of £270. If a personal trainer does three sessions back to back during the exact same time, their net profit would only work out at £105 —almost a third. Furthermore, we must look at the potential for growth. Let's say the coffee shop realises they could sell more units per hour if they had one more member of staff on in the morning. They decide to hire someone, which takes their net profit down from £1.50 to £1.25 per unit sold. However, as a by-product, they're able to increase their units sold from sixty to one hundred per hour during their busiest times. The investment into more staff has now taken net profit from £270 to £375. This has been done without having to risk customer satisfaction through price increases. Our personal trainer, on the other hand, invests in their education and increases their fees by £5 per hour. This takes their hourly net profit (factoring in the cost of the educational course) from £35 to £37.50. The coffee shop was able to increase profit per unit of time by over £100, whereas the personal trainer was only able to do so by £7.50, despite a massive 10% increase in hourly rate (£50 > £55).

Am I suggesting we trade in our tracksuits and protein shakes to become a barista? Well, as much as I enjoy the smell of freshly ground coffee in the morning, I love being a coach and so do you. I'm not saying we should look at alternative careers, I just want to highlight the difficulty in scaling service-based businesses. If you've ever been confused or frustrated about how to make more money in this industry, don't worry. It is a challenging thing do to unless you have distinct objectives. What would sound like a good wage to you? Five years ago, I thought that £6,000 per month was an amazing wage. This works out at delivering twenty-five sessions per week at £60 an hour. That looked straightforward on paper and giving myself five years to achieve this seemed like plenty of time. However, what I wasn't factoring in was net profit. What would I need to do to get myself to that level? Would I need to change working locations to a more affluent area? Would I need to invest heavily in my education and brand? But most importantly, and possibly the most overlooked factor, how would my personal circumstances change in five years' time?

Personal training is in many ways a young person's game. It's quite manageable to earn £2-3,000 a month and work unsociable hours in your early twenties, but this becomes impractical when you have a house, family, and added responsibilities. Some of you may not have any of these right now, but will you in five years? This is why you should start with the future in mind now. Systems to track growth, net profit, outgoings, and scalability of your business are essential for this very reason. Even if you may not have a house and family in five years, you may have saved adequately to launch your own facility or online brand. The reality is, wherever you intend to take yourself in life, it will require an element of financial investment to get you there. You can create this for yourself by starting the building process now.

Rule 5 of Development

Start with the end in mind. Don't think about whether you could sell your business now, imagine you'll be selling it in five years. Have a goal of what you'd like to be earning at that point, then work backwards to see what you need to be improving by each year. Create a systematic process to monitor progress. If you are going to grow a second stream of income, you must ensure that your primary stream is still meeting both growth and profitability, as measured via a quota of sessions per month and bi-annual price increases. As each facet of your business grows, you then have a greater earning potential in the long run. Track everything and have a deliberate model. Once an area becomes self-sufficient, look to see how you can expand in another avenue. If you can show how you came to create your wealth, you have an extremely potent formula for continuing your success. All this needs to be analysed and monitored in a manner so that it could be easily presented to a critical business conglomerate.

Don't be afraid to grow slowly and proportionally to what your business (you) can manage. It is essential that you see the wood through the trees. Never underestimate the power of making small, quantifiable improvements over time. Approach your finances just like you would improving your physique. One kilo of lean muscle on and 1% of body fat down in a year doesn't seem like a lot, but how will your physique look if you do this consistently for five years straight. Furthermore, what's to prevent you from doing this the rest of your career?

END NOTE
WHAT IS WEALTH?

I'd like to end by discussing a concept that is extremely important for you to consider going forward. This idea will be dissected so that we see it from both a practical and personal perspective. I want you to think about wealth and what it means to you, not just from a financial point of view, but from a personal fulfilment aspect as well.

Would earning £10,000 per month make you wealthy? Your financial wealth is only proportional to your diligence in spending and saving. It doesn't matter how much you earn, if you don't put it away and have financial responsibility, you'll always be confused as to why you're not progressing in life. Financial freedom will make your personal growth a much easier process. However, you don't have to be exceedingly wealthy to be financially free. Wealth is the ability to create abundance of a desirable commodity. You are only wealthy if you know how to amass more than you expend. One of the biggest dangers of increasing your income is exponentially driving up your outgoings in tandem. It's important that you learn to respect money and constantly save for a project on a larger scale. As you grow, your ability to earn money will grow. You'll see the value in marginal gains and the power of patience mixed with a long-term plan. Your ability to do anything in life will be potentiated by funding; therefore, it's essential to learn how to create this funding yourself. Be your own investor. It makes the satisfaction of achieving a long-term goal even sweeter.

Right now, I'd like you to make a commitment to start saving money. I'd like you to call this money your five-year plan fund. At the end of each month, take 5% of what you were paid or generated that month and put it in to a separate bank account. I don't want you to draw any money out of this account for five years. The reason for this is simple. If someone were to give you £7,500–10,000 now, what would you do with it? Would you invest in education? Your own facility? A house deposit maybe? For many people reading this, that is a substantial amount of money to receive in one go. Why not give it to yourself in five years? You have the ability to make your life either easy or hard for yourself. As trainers, our biggest fear is lack of certainty and direction. The goal of charging £50 an hour, earning £6,000 a month, and having £10,000 waiting for you in a pot in half a decade's time gives you both a purpose and clear goal. These aren't just the necessary elements for long-term business success; they're the essential ingredients for happiness as well.

Whilst seeking wealth, you must always remind yourself of the bigger picture. Financial wealth is only one element of true fulfilment. Just like you can't neglect a muscle group from a well-rounded physique, you can't neglect other aspects of your life such as health, happiness, relationships, relaxation, and spirituality. If you do, you are not wealthy, you just have a lot of money. This raises the question, what do you need all this money for?

One of the biggest things I want you to take away from *The 5 x 5 Rule* is the concept of lifestyle design. Yes, hard work is important, but you should never work so hard that it's to the detriment of your family life, health, and mental wellbeing. You are much better off working as smart as you do hard in the world of health and fitness. I don't want people to feel frustrated by this industry anymore. I don't want people to feel like they're not being valued or taken seriously. My goal is to open each coach's eyes to the fact that they have complete control over their earnings, time, and development. This job can be as lucrative as it is rewarding if you have a deliberate and thought-out model.

If I were to talk about balance, this would make me a hypocrite. Nothing of great excellence is born through balance. You need uneven distributions of effort to excel in one area and it would be naive to believe otherwise. This being said, many assume that unrelenting hard work and sacrifice must be adhered to for weeks, months, and years to achieve success. This isn't the case. Your progress can be measured objectively by tasks completed and income generated. This gives you data. Data never lie. If you aren't getting through the tasks that need to be completed, you don't need to work harder, you need to be more efficient with your time. Don't count the hours that you work, make the hours that you work count. Never let the feeling of needing to develop come between the truest riches we have in life. If you do not take time out on a daily basis to talk, laugh, or play with someone dear to you, no amount of money in the world will make you wealthy. By focusing only on finances, you have completely missed the point of *The 5 x 5 Rule*. This book is designed to help you purchase the most valuable currency there is: time. You must use your new-found systems and surplus of income to can create memories and security for the ones closest to you. My wife text me one morning saying our six year old daughter had done her hair on her own for the first time and that she was extremely proud of herself. When I got home I joked with her and said "Well done, I will give you one million pounds in pocket money". She shook her head and said "Can you play with me instead?" Children will always remind you of what's really important in life. We are all much richer than we think, we just get distracted by thinking otherwise. You can create immense levels of fulfilment through the things that cost nothing at all.

I would like to sincerely thank you for purchasing this book. It was an absolute pleasure to write and I wish you tremendous success in building your business, increasing your income and improving the lives of others

Made in the USA
Monee, IL
10 August 2022

11352186R00146